Adding Insult to Injury

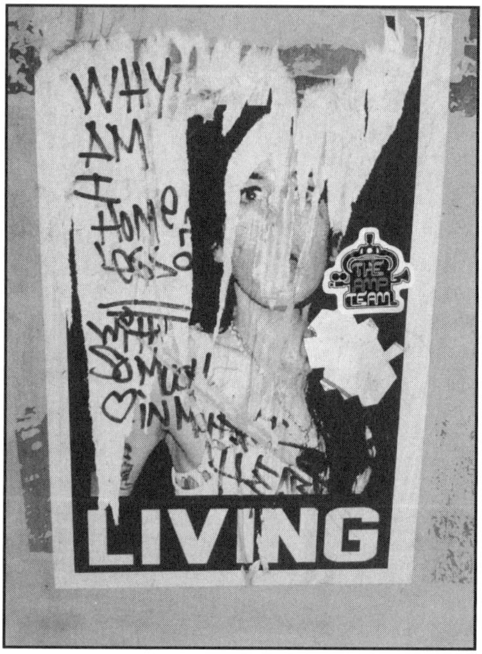

Why Am I Homeless
with So Much Love in My Heart

Adding Insult to Injury

(Mis)Treating Homeless Women in Our Mental Health System

Laura Huey
Rose Ricciardelli

LYNNE RIENNER PUBLISHERS
BOULDER
LONDON

Published in the United States of America in 2016 by
Lynne Rienner Publishers, Inc.
1800 30th Street, Boulder, Colorado 80301
www.rienner.com

and in the United Kingdom by
Lynne Rienner Publishers, Inc.
3 Henrietta Street, Covent Garden, London WC2E 8LU

Library of Congress Cataloging-in-Publication Data
Names: Huey, Laura, author. | Ricciardelli, Rose, 1979– author.
Title: Adding insult to injury : (mis) treating homeless women in our mental health system / by Laura Huey and Rose Ricciardelli.
Description: Boulder, Colorado : Lynne Rienner Publishers, Inc., 2016. | Includes bibliographical references.
Identifiers: LCCN 2016003976 | ISBN 9781626375611 (hc : alk. paper)
Subjects: LCSH: Homeless women—Mental health. | Homeless women—Mental health services.
Classification: LCC RC451.4.H64 H84 2016 | DDC 362.2/0425086942—dc23
LC record available at http://lccn.loc.gov/2016003976.

British Cataloguing in Publication Data
A Cataloguing in Publication record for this book is available from the British Library.

Printed and bound in the United States of America

The paper used in this publication meets the requirements of the American National Standard for Permanence of Paper for Printed Library Materials Z39.48-1992.

5 4 3 2 1

Contents

1

Homeless Women and Mental Health

Laura meets Nikki while interviewing her friend, Kesha. Laura and Kesha have been sitting in a small counseling room in one of the shelters that dot San Pedro Street in Los Angeles's Skid Row District. Laura is asking Kesha, a victim of childhood abuse, a series of questions about her experiences of trauma and the coping strategies she uses to deal with the effects of what she has been through when they hear a knock at the door. Opening it, Laura finds Nikki, an African American woman in her late thirties, standing on the other side, politely letting her know that she is waiting to be interviewed next. Hearing her friend's voice, Kesha speaks up and asks if Nikki could join the discussion.

Both women have become homeless for financial reasons and are desperate to move out of the shelter and out of Skid Row. Nikki has just started a job and begins to describe what getting up in the morning and leaving Skid Row for her new job are like.

NIKKI: I have to be at work at six o'clock in the morning. I get up at four o'clock in the morning, so I'm up when the action starts on the streets. So I see people knocking on people's tents for heroin. I'm standing at the bus stop, you see so much. You hear women prostituting their daughters out. Are you serious? This is like real? It's like a bad movie.

LAURA: How does it feel to be the odd person out?

KESHA: [laughing] It's weird!

NIKKI: It's crazy! Because what's normal here is not normal anywhere else. . . . It's like a bizarre world. Like on Seinfeld. Everything that was normal, the rules don't apply here!

Both found life at the shelter stressful, and each was coping with the fights, the drama, and the strange rules in different ways. Kesha, who had been diagnosed as borderline obsessive compulsive disorder (OCD), acknowledged that her recently developed daily cleaning rituals served a dual purpose: they kept her area free of scabies, lice, and bedbugs, and they permitted her a measure of control within a space in which she had none. Leaning in slightly, she explained, "You can't control the situation you're in, but you can keep your locker clean, [and] you can keep your bed straight." Nikki was struggling with feelings of depression and anxiety over her situation: "My crazy is me being a single parent and having my daughter down here. She's twenty-three. It's a control issue of . . . my eating's out of control. I can't control nothing around me, but I can control if I put some chips and some cheesecake in me." When the discussion turned to other methods of coping, the subject of antidepressants came up, and Nikki said that "especially here" (indicating the shelter) pharmacological solutions for any problems were commonly recommended by staff and the shelter's doctor. Whereas Kesha had already seen a psychiatrist at a local clinic and been prescribed the antidepressant sertraline to deal with her anxiety issues,[1] Nikki's case manager at the shelter recommended she take antidepressants, going so far as to refer Nikki to the shelter's doctor in order to secure a prescription.

NIKKI: They wanted to give me some Zoloft.
KESHA: That's what they tried to give me!
NIKKI: And something else.
LAURA: Who did you go see? Your doctor?
NIKKI: My case manager. She was referring me to the doctor here.
LAURA: To then get on the . . .
NIKKI: Zoloft.
LAURA: What was your response?
NIKKI: I was like that's not what I was coming here for. My whole thing was to make sense of all of this. I'm gonna be honest with you. I'm thirty-eight years old. My intention in life was never *ever* to live on Skid Row. [Everyone starts laughing.] I'm just keeping it real. I just need to make it make sense. It didn't make sense.
LAURA: Have you had an opportunity to do any one-on-one counseling?
NIKKI: Actually, I have with [names a counselor]. She's good. She really helps me put a perspective . . . she really helps me see the other side. That's what I needed. I didn't need a pill. I just needed some therapy.

Nikki's story is not unusual. Over the years we have come to realize there are thousands and thousands of Nikkis, homeless or otherwise impoverished women who are struggling to make sense of, and to hopefully overcome, events in their lives that sometimes defy ready explanation. When they seek help, they are frequently directed to a mental health system that, arguably, all too often opts for pharmaceutical over therapeutic interventions. It tells them the solution is pills that neurochemically alter the brain instead of also addressing cognitive needs as a potential solution. As in the case of Nikki, such views not only predominate within the healthcare system itself but are shared by those who work within the institutions that frequently structure the lives of homeless citizens: shelters, public social work offices, courts, and jails.

As we will show in the subsequent chapters, lacking few alternate resources, if any, and variously persuaded, compelled, bribed, and coerced into accepting this form of treatment as the solution to their problems, untold numbers of women find themselves dealing with the effects of trauma and chronic stressors by chemically burying them. Although relying on placebo effects and sedation is presumably cheaper in the short term than providing expensive therapeutic sessions like psychotherapy and secure housing, the reality is simple: for many women, the underlying issues remain, and thus the lives of too few women ever improve.

The Argument

Despite the definition of the World Health Organization (WHO) of health as a "state of complete physical, mental, and social well-being and not merely the absence of disease and infirmity" (Armstrong and Armstrong 2010, p. 4), over the past several decades a notable shift has occurred in how societies think about individuals' well-being, a shift away from ensuring the physical, social, and mental health of citizens. This shift is attributable to a combination of factors, including the reliance on the medicine model (e.g., a variation of the allopathic model), the medicalization of common conditions, and the associated stigma, as well as the resulting ascendancy of a model of human cognition, emotions, and behavior that purports to answer all questions about why humans are the way they are: biopsychiatry.[2] The US healthcare system is based in the for-profit sector and utilizes predominantly an allopathic approach to healthcare, which is focused on penetrating the body physically (surgery) or chemically (drugs) as a means for curing what professionals in this area see as illness and ill health (Armstrong and Armstrong 2010). The system has become jaded due to the motivations of private institutions (e.g., pharmaceutical companies) that add to the for-profit model as they dominate and control the progression of medicine in a quest for monetary gain. Together these factors dictate the way in which healthcare is delivered and its impact on individual experiences and views of healthcare as an institution, again as a means of promoting the continuation of the allopathic approach to healthcare.

The allopathic medical model emerged in the nineteenth century as the primary medical model in the Western world. *Allopathy*, a combination of *allos*, meaning "opposite," and *pathos*, meaning "suffering," was coined by the German physician C. F. S. Hahnemann (1755–1843) in reference to the seemingly barbaric medical practices common to the eighteenth century, such as bloodletting, purging, and toxic drugs.[3] The idea behind such practices was tied to the notion of treating conditions based on their "opposite," a reality common even now in Western medicine where, for example, constipation is treated with a laxative or a headache with a drug designed to eliminate the headache, such that "cuts and chemicals" remain predominant treatment options for illness (Jarvis 1996; Kaufman 1988). As Stephen Lyng explains,

> [the] medical perception focuses on the problem of discovering the objective conditions that give rise to the subjective sensations that we know as patient complaints (defined as symptoms in this system). In other words, the problem is to objectify the subjective sensations of the patient. This task is accomplished by translating all illness (i.e., the patient's subjective sense of abnormality) into disease. (1990, pp. 102–103)

Not surprisingly, in general, the medical model discounts alternative approaches to healthcare, such as chiropractic and homeopathic medicine, which are rarely seen as actual medicine or cures for illness or poor health. Indeed, Western society over the years has ingrained assumptions regarding health and healthcare, limiting alternative medical practices. These assumptions are simply viewed as societal truths. For example, one so-called truth is that illness is biological, a truth that in turn disregards the social determinants of health that focus on the impact that environment, socioeconomic status, or standards of living can have on physical and mental health (Armstrong and Armstrong 2010). Indeed, these social determinants cannot be disregarded in their role in shaping the psychological health and well-being of homeless women.

Unquestionably, however, the allopathic medical model has saved many lives, and the resulting advancements in medicine have increased life expectancy in North America (Armstrong and Armstrong 2010). However, rather than trying to take preventive measures, the focus on science, biology, medical advancement, and cures highlights the political economy and consumerism underlying the current healthcare system, essentially, orienting it toward the pursuit of profit (Armstrong and Armstrong 2010). In the United States, this system is shaped by private institutions (e.g., doctors, pharmaceutical companies) that add to the for-profit sector. Institutions dominate and control the progression of medicine; therefore, many scholars argue, developments and innovations (new medications, new healthcare practices, and new medical devices) are no longer a means of responding to the needs of society but instead represent the quest for monetary gain, power, and resources (Armstrong and Armstrong 2010). Political ideologies that have shaped governance provide a fertile breeding ground for the progression of individual health advocacy wherein patients who can afford to do so pursue their own health needs. They act as consumers of healthcare and advocate on behalf of their own needs and desires. The question then becomes, what is a healthcare need?

In 1992, Peter Conrad and Joseph Schneider drew attention to a new trend: the transformation of what some saw as deviance and other social problems into medical problems. In essence, they argue that, within this new paradigm, "deviance" is relabeled as "illness," and the individual comes to be viewed as someone who can be helped, even cured, by medical authorities and their technical knowledge. Through this process, termed *medicalization*, the patient becomes largely disempowered, falling under the authority of medical professionals. Although we do not take this position, some scholars go so far as to argue that mental illness does not exist but is instead a label that has been successfully applied to particular body processes and social problems (see Bowden 2014; Conrad and Barker, 2010; Fried et al. 2015; Hesslow 1993; Launer 2014; Pickersgill 2013). As such, all medical facts are argued to be socially created products, arguably constructed and developed by interested parties and claims makers with much to gain, that allow medicine to reign as an institution of social control (Conrad and Barker 2010).

Medicalization occurs at three levels: the conceptual level, where medical vocabulary is used to define the problem; the institutional level, where medical personnel supervise treatment or act as gatekeepers to treatment; and the interactional level, which is the point at which doctors treat what they see as the medical problems of their patients (Armstrong and Armstrong 2010). At each level, relationships of power situate what is labeled as the treatment of the patients, whose agency is by and large dictated by their adherence to the medical directives put forth by the medical professionals from whom they are receiving care. Thus, with medicalization, not only do increasingly common problems become redefined as manifestations of psychopathology requiring intervention, but individuals grappling with an issue are left to seek out and then adhere to a prescribed course of care if they want to be viewed as helping themselves and their situation. Conrad and Schneider (1992) explained that by being reclassified as patients, rather than just seen as homeless women, individuals become entitled to help, but they are first put into the submissive position of adherence if they are to get help or to "rectify their situation" under the medical profession.

Within the medical model is where biopsychiatry falls. At its root, biopsychiatry is a worldview predicated on the belief that human suffering can be grouped into discrete categories based on symptomology, labeled as clinical disorders, and then linked to dysfunctional biological processes within the nervous system. This perspective continues despite the fact, again evidenced in more recent criticisms of the *Diagnostic and Statistical Manual of Mental Disorders* (DSM-V), that little evidence can be given for specific biological markers of mental illness (see Pickersgill 2013). An individual's problems, as suggested by biopsychiatry, are not caused by environmental factors (e.g., social determinants of health); rather, the root of problems and thus the potential solutions lie in the functioning of neurons and synapses, as dictated by genes. According to this paradigm, these processes can be beneficially altered through expert administration of neurochemical compounds that inhibit or reverse the effects of malfunctioning neurons and synapses—the so-called chemical imbalances of the brain—through selective or nondiscriminate chemical actions. Said another way, a reliance on drugs by medical professionals, specifically prescription medications designed to alter the functioning of the brain, underlies biopsychiatry. The administration of these drugs is the province of a growing number of practitioners within the so-called helping professions in the United States—psychiatrists, primary care doctors, nurse practitioners, and pharmacists—who not only are sanctioned to diagnose conditions but have been granted prescriptive authority and thus the privilege to treat patients using psychoactive substances.[4] However, we are not suggesting all prescribing is unnecessary, erroneous, or inappropriate; instead, here we point to where prescriptions replace rather than accompany therapeutic interventions or serve as ineffective or lazy Band-Aid approaches targeting overrepresented populations, like homeless women.[5]

Much has already been written about the growing biopsychiatrization of everyday life and the accompanying neurochemicals biopsychiatric practitioners deploy (Bentall 2009; Frances 2013; Greenberg 2013; Rimke and Brock 2012). Indeed, a veritable cottage industry has sprung up to warn citizens of the risks found in converting everyday behaviors into mental health problems, giving our children drugs for behavior problems,[6] or relying too heavily on antidepressants to make us, if not happy, then at least momentarily content. Although much has already been said about this medicalization, and more specifically biopsychiatrization, in relation to the general public, one area of social life can be examined in which biopsychiatry wields an enormous power that is seldom scrutinized and generally accepted as both right and necessary, that is, in the lives of homeless citizens.

Long considered a repository of any and all social ills, homelessness has been transformed from a social space within which individuals appear as morally corrupt degenerates to one holding an ever-increasing assortment of individuals deemed mentally ill. This change is easily explained. Psychiatry, as embedded in the medical sector of society, has long been associated with homelessness as providing both an explanation and potential cure for this state. With respect to the former, a significant body of commentary attributes the character of contemporary homelessness to the move away from asylums and other psychiatric residential treatment facilities toward community-based forms of treatment (see, for example, Dear and Wolch 1987). Thus, the ranks of homeless citizens today are said to be largely drawn from those who were previously institutionalized, or who would have been institutionalized today if such facilities were still routinely used in this way.[7]

Having redefined this social problem as psychiatric in origin within a larger social framework that increasingly views the biopsychiatric worldview as providing the solution to most, if not all, of society's complex and mundane problems, one can see how biopsychiatry has been touted as the solution to homelessness and how unstintingly faith is to be placed in the chemical regimens often prescribed. This unwavering faith has had important consequences for how homeless citizens are treated. It has spawned new ways of thinking about, and responding to, their problems, which, on the surface, appear similar to how society views the problems of other segments of the population. Invoking a disease metaphor to explain the causes of their distress, homeless citizens learn their only hope is to participate in the treatment of their "chemical imbalances." Within this framework, responsibilized self-care is portrayed as an individually empowering act; however, as we shall discuss, it is ultimately one that does little more than maintain social and structural inequities that disempower individuals who are suffering.

Thus far we have focused on the history of the medical model in the United States and, more specifically, on the way in which biopsychiatric power manifests at a macro level, a theme to which we return in the following chapter. Our primary interest, however, is in analyzing its effects on individuals, a task that reveals three principal forms of biopsychiatric power, that we use to refer to—the power of professionals to diagnose, prescribe, and garner compliance with drug treatment regimes, and the way this power manifests in the lives of people who are homeless. The first power is that of the authority to diagnose individual suffering, giving it a name and an ascribed cause as well as redefining the individual through the application of a diagnostic label. No longer simply Jane or

Joe, the individual is endowed with a new institutional and sometimes personal identity as a "bipolar" patient or as a "schizophrenic." The second form of power we discuss here is the power to prescribe a course of treatment based on a diagnosed condition. To the extent that the underlying problem is deemed biochemical in nature, this prescriptive power is enacted through instructing patients to routinely ingest one or more psychiatric drugs that are deemed necessary to right their perceived chemical imbalance. The third power we analyze here is the ability to garner individual compliance with psychiatric drug prescriptions through a variety of persuasive and coercive techniques. These techniques, as will be made evident, work both directly through community-based programs, institutional confinement, and forced outpatient treatment and also indirectly through networks of alliances with other institutions.

Further tying these three principal forms of power together is how they are easily forced upon people in psychological distress or living in a state of homelessness—people who are stigmatized (Goffman 1963). Erving Goffman defines stigma as "an attribute that is deeply discrediting . . . a relation[ship] between stereotype and attribute" (1963, p. 4). Stereotypes, per Goffman, originate and are established in society, whereas attributes are characteristics possessed by a person. Stereotypes and attributes are related in that when an attribute is stigmatized, the stigma suggests the bearer possesses an othering quality that qualifies that person for social rejection, exclusion, or isolation. Stigma defines the bearer's master status and as such structures that person's self-perceptions, interactions, and the social order (Goffman 1963). It creates divisions among community members across societies.

The stigma experienced by the homeless women in our study is multifaceted and complex. They are stigmatized by their cognitive state (mental illness), their homelessness, and even their ethnicity or race, sexuality, or criminal past. The relationships between such attributes and the associated stereotypes shape their lived experiences, including opportunities available, treatment by others, and even self-perceptions (Kondrat and Early 2011). In consequence, bearing a stigma and the associated label ensures that their esteem is low, that they live with the knowledge that they will be judged simply by the fact that they reside on Skid Row and they will be rejected by others (Kondrat and Early 2011). Stigma, always a dynamic process and never a static reality, places these women in an inferior position by focusing on their virtual social identity rather than on their actual social identity (Goffman 1963), consequently leaving them subordinate and disempowered. In this same context, the stigma and associated prejudice, even discrimination, these women face leave them even more vulnerable to those with biopsychiatric power, or any position endowed with power due to having the resources these women need given their desperate need (see Chapter 2).

We stress here that the problems of homeless citizens are not trivial or unworthy of assistance. Indeed, as discussed in Chapter 3, the vast majority of homeless individuals live under the weight of the emotional and mental scars they carry as a result of living trauma-infused lives. As a consequence of their histories of abandonment, neglect, violence, and deprivation, among a host of other tragedies, a significant number of homeless persons develop trauma-induced responses that are recoded as symptoms of psychiatric conditions. With few, if any, resources available to them, individuals are placed within a system that is often completely ineffective at recognizing and responding appropriately to the effects of trauma. Indeed, typical treatment responses to issues of trauma often entail little more than outmoded forms of talk therapy (Huey, Fthenos, and Hryniewicz 2012), prescriptions for psychoactive drugs, or both. When individuals do not respond to what the system defines as treatment, as is often the case, such failures are easily attributed to the individuals—their so-called disease being treatment resistant—and not to ineffective treatment or relationships with the treatment provider that may bar treatment effectiveness. Homeless citizens will then cycle in and out of the various institutions that make up the circuits of control in which homeless citizens are routinely plugged: shelters, hospitals, jails, and prisons. Of course, these spaces too carry a stigma of their own, which further burdens the women who must somehow navigate these realities and the associated meanings their experiences suggest to members of society. Not surprisingly, as these women increasingly fail to improve in their ability to function in ways society sees as normal, the role of psychiatric drugs becomes even more crucial to their management, both within the community and behind institutional walls. This book, in response, is about society's failure to provide adequate mental health care for homeless citizens, the majority of whom are deeply traumatized and stigmatized and experience chronic distress as a consequence. This failure, we argue, can be traced to the rise of the discourse of biopsychiatry, which has become the dominant lens through which homelessness and its attendant ills have come to be viewed (Rose 1998). Reliance on this lens has led professionals to turn away from the healing of trauma in favor of an overreliance on psychiatric drugs to suppress the purported dysfunctions of those least able to resist biopsychiatric power. In essence, then, what we describe here is not healing but the expedient management of problems, from the problems of individuals to the supposed social plight of so-called problem populations.

The Focus

Little doubt can be found that biopsychiatric power is a set of processes, embedded in the allopathic medical model, with the potential to affect all homeless citizens who come into contact with the institutions that make up or support the mental health complex (i.e., shelters, courts, hospitals, jails, and prisons). Indeed, these institutions bear a stigma of their own—the prison, the asylum, the court—that in itself is indicative of the empowerment of those with authority in such facilities. The doctor holds authority over the patient, the prison officer over the prisoner, and the judge over the defendant. The patient, prisoner, defendant, and so on, are known by their master status (Goffman 1963): the label they hold evinces their disempowerment and leaves them susceptible to what is put forth by those in positions of authority as "for her own good" (Ehrenreich and English 2005). With this situation in mind, we made the focus of this book women who are homeless and the way their responses to trauma come to be redefined as forms of psychopathology to be treated principally, if not solely, through the administration of psychoactive drugs—chemicals—without the accompaniment of any counseling, treatment, or trauma-informed care. We have chosen to narrow the scope of this book in this fashion because of the unique vulnerabilities experienced by homeless women as a group (see Chapter 3).

To illustrate why women might be more likely to be subject to biopsychiatric powers, we begin by examining the link between gender and trauma. Without intending to diminish men's experiences of trauma, we note that studies have consistently found significant gender-based differences in exposure to forms of trauma and the responses they generate. Although men may typically be exposed to a greater number of potentially traumatizing events, in the form of accidents, combat, and physical assaults (Norris, Foster, and Weisshaar 2002), women are more likely to experience interpersonal violence, particularly involving someone they trust (child abuse, sexual assault, and domestic violence being three notable examples) (Ghafoori, Barragan, and Palinkas 2013; Tolin and Foa 2006). Women have also been found to experience greater levels of posttraumatic distress. For example, in a meta-analysis of studies of gender, trauma, and posttraumatic stress disorder (PTSD) symptomology, David Tolin and Edna Foa (2006) found that women exposed to trauma were more likely than men to report symptoms of mental distress by a ratio of approximately two to one. Women also reported higher levels of traumatic flashbacks, avoidance behaviors, and stress arousal (Ditlevsen and Elklit 2010), which last for a longer duration than found among traumatized males (Breslau et al. 1999). Women also appear to be at increased risk of postevent depression (Ghafoori, Barragan, and Palinkas 2013; Tolin and Foa 2006). One theory put forward to explain these differences suggests that women's exposure to interpersonal violence by those they trust—caregivers, intimate partners—is more emotionally and psychologically devastating because of the element of betrayal involved in such actions (Freyd 1994; Hetzel-Riggin and Roby 2013), and that such betrayals threaten their sense of safety and security in profound ways (Janoff-Bulman 1992). Others point to the fact that of the various forms of traumatic experience analyzed by researchers, sexual assault, which is reported with greater frequency by women, is also associated with the highest reported rates of PTSD (Tang and Freyd 2012).

Regardless of the underlying dynamics, one thing remains clear: women exposed to traumatizing events, overall, are at an increased risk of developing symptoms of mental and emotional distress. The fact remains that women make up only a small percentage of the homeless population yet suffer from many vulnerabilities, particularly in ways unique to women. Thus, if women are generally more vulnerable in this regard, then the expectation is to see homeless women, who experience high rates of violence and significant life stressors and often live in highly adverse conditions, as being at substantial risk of developing or experiencing worsening mental health conditions (Davies-Netzley, Hurlburt, and Hough 1996; D'Ercole and Streuning 1990; Huey, Fthenos, and Hryniewicz 2012; Jasinski et al. 2010; Lam and Rosenheck 1998; Larney et al. 2009). And, of course, that is exactly what researchers have consistently noted. In a meta-analysis of research conducted in the 1990s, Marjorie Robertson and Marilyn Winkleby found that homeless women report higher levels of distress than that found in the general population, and they also consistently report higher levels of mental health problems:

> The lifetime rates of schizophrenia in homeless women ranged from 2.5 to 17.1%, compared to 1.7% for women in the general population. Rates of major depression ranged from 15.8 to 32% compared to 10.2% for women in the general population. Bipolar disorders ranged from 3.3 to 12% compared to less than 1% in the general population. (1996, p. 317)

More recently, Angela Hudson and her colleagues reviewed the literature on victimization among homeless citizens, observing that childhood sexual abuse and physical violence are generally associated "with poor general health and psychiatric co-morbidities, including post-traumatic stress disorder, depression, and suicidal ideation" (2010, p. 1215). In their study of experiences of adult assault among homeless women, the authors found links between physical abuse and depressive symptoms, including loneliness, low self-esteem, and social withdrawal (Hudson et al, 2010; see also Ambrosio et al. 1992). One longitudinal study found that "childhood sexual abuse, living in a shelter, physical violence, childhood physical abuse, and death or injury of a friend or relative predicted avoidant coping and symptoms of depression" among homeless women (Rayburn et al. 2005, p. 667). Perhaps it is not entirely surprising to find that to deal with the distressing psychological and emotional effects of trauma, many impoverished women turn to forms of avoidant coping, including drugs and alcohol (Rayburn et al. 2005; Robertson and Winkleby 1996; Yeater et al. 2010).

In general, not only do women report higher levels of mental distress following a traumatizing event (Koopmans and Lamers 2007), but they also appear more willing to use mental health services (Andrews, Issakidis, and Carter 2001; Rhodes et al. 2002; Sorenson and Siegel 1992; Wang et al. 2005). This finding appears to apply equally to homeless women: despite the fact that impoverished women face barriers to accessing healthcare services, researchers suggest a number of women do seek treatment for mental health issues (Huey, Fthenos, and Hryniewicz 2012; Tam, Zlotnick, and Bradley 2008). In one study, almost a quarter of the sample of 663 impoverished female participants had sought mental health treatment after a traumatic experience (Rayburn et al. 2005). By way of contrast, in a study of mental service use among homeless men, researchers found that "men are often reluctant to ask for help," and those surveyed were "not likely to seek help for their physical and psychological struggles" (Amato and Macdonald 2011, p. 227).

Their increased use of healthcare services provides women a greater number of opportunities to be diagnosed with a psychiatric condition and offered drugs as treatment. With respect to the general population, this supposition is borne out by studies of prescription drug use that reveal higher rates of psychiatric drug use among women (Hausken et al. 2010; Hausken, Skurtveit, and Tverdal, 2007; Medco 2011; Roe, McNamara, and Motheral 2002). Data from one of the major pharmacy benefit managers in the United States shows a similar pattern: "Women are far more likely to take a drug to treat a mental health condition than men, with more than a quarter of the adult female population on these drugs in 2010 as compared to 15 percent of men" (Medco 2011, p. 2). According to the Medco (2011) study, women were more likely than men to use antidepressants (men's usage in this category is almost half that of women), antianxiety drugs (again, women's rate of use is nearly twice that of men), and to be prescribed antipsychotics. The only category where males exceed females in drug use is with respect to stimulants prescribed for attention deficit hyperactivity disorder (ADHD). Even here, girls are catching up, with rates of prescriptions for girls described as increasing by almost 40 percent over ten years. These findings are mirrored elsewhere. In relation to antianxiety drugs, one set of Norwegian studies found that "being a woman" was a significant predictor of antianxiety drug use (Hausken et al. 2010, p. 472), with women being twice as likely to use these drugs as men (Hausken, Skurtveit, and Tverdal 2007).

In relation to psychiatric drug prescription and usage among homeless women, researchers know almost nothing. Despite high rates of reported psychiatric diagnoses within homeless communities (Austin, Anderson, and Gelberg 2008; Bassuk et al. 1998; Larney et al. 2009), treatment issues generally and the use of psychiatric drug treatment in particular have failed to generate broader attention from researchers beyond issues of drug efficacy and treatment compliance. Thus, one cannot say with any degree of certainty whether homeless women are more likely to be prescribed and consume psychiatric drugs than their male counterparts. However, theorizing their greater use in the population is not unreasonable given everything currently known about the gendered nature of mental health issues in both homeless communities and larger society.

To summarize our reasons for having narrowed the focus of this book to examining the range of homeless women's experiences with mental illness: to the extent that homeless women experience relatively high rates of trauma, are significantly more likely to be emotionally and psychologically affected by trauma, and are more likely to visit a healthcare provider in search of treatment, they represent a group that is more likely to be recast as exhibiting any number of forms of mental illness. Further, this mental illness is then seen as amenable to treatment with drugs, especially psychoactive drugs. Thus, although this tendency cannot be seen as solely a gendered phenomenon, it *is* highly gendered. Further support for this contention comes from a review of the history of the "psy sciences," a term we borrow from Nikolas Rose (1998), a domain notoriously littered with examples of how women's suffering has been pathologized and their bodies subjected to harrowing treatments (Tasca et al. 2012).

Sources

The inspiration for our desire to explore the lives of homeless women came from a series of interactions we had while conducting research on trauma and coping mechanisms. The impetus for the current study can be traced back to Detroit and Chicago, where the research team, led by Laura Huey, conducted in-depth qualitative interviews with almost 100 women. A further fifty-five interviews were then conducted with female participants in Liverpool and Manchester in the hope of teasing out a comparative approach to services. In the early days of the research, the focus was specifically on trauma, access to mental health services, and service usage. Although many of the women interviewed had participated in various forms of counseling, few spoke directly of experiences with psychiatry or of being prescribed psychiatric drugs. However, various women were encountered who, if they did not speak directly about their encounters with psychiatry, manifested physical signs of such encounters in the form of visible side effects of psychiatric drug use.

In 2012 the decision was made to relocate the fieldwork to Los Angeles, a city with a sizable homeless population that would afford greater opportunities to locate female participants. In shifting research sites, we also opted to expand the scope of the research to include a more broadly defined set of coping strategies that women use to deal with the effects of trauma. The current study is based on these interviews, which yielded significant insights into the use of psychiatric drugs to treat women's problems and, in particular, the way prescription drugs were being used in some cases as a means of modifying women's behaviors. During the first round of research in Los Angeles, the research team collected 107 interviews that were subsequently transcribed and analyzed. The initial results highlighted something that had been brewing in the back of our minds since starting this work: the great extent to which psychiatric drugs were being used routinely and often exclusively for the treatment of symptoms of trauma-based distress. Whereas the women in Detroit and Chicago seldom spoke of using psychiatric drugs, perhaps from fears of being stigmatized or because few had the opportunity to see a psychiatrist or general practitioner, women in Los Angeles were much more forthcoming about their experiences with both medical professionals and their psychoactive solutions. As a result, when we returned for two more rounds of interviews, the focus continued to remain on broader issues of trauma and coping, but more time was now spent listening to women's experiences of their encounters with such professionals. Within this phase of the interviews, women had much to tell us about the mental health diagnoses they had received, their feelings about the various forms of therapy they had tried, the treatments they had been prescribed, treatment compliance issues, and so on. In total, the team conducted 201 ($n = 201$)[8] interviews in Los Angeles.[9]

The Shape of Things to Come

We have organized the chapters of this book to follow the lines of our argument. Thus, Chapter 2 provides a conceptual framework by introducing some of the relevant literature on structural violence, the medicalization of social conditions, and stigma. Specifically we explore these phenomena in relation to how biopsychiatry as a worldview has come to dominate cultural discussions of human functioning and human suffering. We then investigate how homelessness has become medicalized, and we look at, in further detail, the role of biopsychiatry in the social response to homelessness, from the psychiatrization of the problem of homelessness in the 1980s to the use of psychoactive drugs to treat symptoms and regulate behaviors. We conclude the chapter with a critique of the medicalized and biopsych account of homelessness, providing an alternative, trauma-based explanation for the signs of emotional and psychological distress seen in homeless populations.

In support of our contention that trauma is a significant factor in the lives of homeless women, the nature of the suffering experienced by study participants is the focus of Chapter 3. Drawing on the women's own words, we break the first half of this chapter into three parts, which detail, in turn, the traumatic experiences women have faced in childhood and adulthood, as well as the struggles associated with becoming and being homeless. The discussion then turns to the damaging psychological effects of these experiences and how women attempt to cope with few available resources.

The purpose of Chapter 4 is to detail the first of the three forms of biopsychiatric power previously enumerated: the defining of women's problems through the act of diagnosis. We begin by exploring how women came to receive psychiatric treatment and the means by which psychiatrists, general practitioners, and other medical professionals translate women's suffering into a mental health diagnosis. Then, continuing to draw on participant experiences, we examine some of the diagnoses women had received, contextualizing these diagnoses by situating them in relation to the types of suffering women had experienced. We also consider individual thoughts and feelings about diagnoses, including the extent to which individuals self-identified with the labels affixed to their suffering.

Chapter 5 examines the second form of biopsychiatric power detailed here: the ability of medical professionals to prescribe psychoactive drug treatment for their patients, drugs that can null or suppress effects in terms of their emotional, cognitive, and behavioral functioning. First, we look at the types of psychiatric drugs that women in the Los Angeles study were prescribed, before turning to an examination of how women viewed the effects of these drugs. As our analysis reveals, for some, psychiatric drugs are seen as vehicles for self-improvement: that is, as solutions to the physical, mental, spiritual, social, existential, and other problems they face. One of these solutions, and perhaps the most obvious, is through symptom abatement. However, emphasis is also placed by some on the use of psychoactive drugs as part of their reform-oriented work: that is, as a means of altering one's feelings and cognitions in the hope of effecting permanent life changes. We also consider the views of those who have alternative perspectives on the use of psychiatric drugs, views shaped either through beliefs in alternative healing systems or as a result of observing or experiencing null or negative effects from these drugs.

The focus of Chapter 6 is the third manifestation of biopsychiatric power in homeless communities: the range of persuasive (soft) and coercive (hard) techniques employed within and across institutions to garner treatment compliance. In particular, we explore the institutional environments within which psychiatric drug treatment decisions are made, supported, and enforced. Forms of persuasion include, for example, community-based programs that reinforce what is seen as patient responsibility in pill taking. When persuasion fails, various coercive mechanisms also can be deployed in order to enforce treatment compliance. These range from soft coercion in community treatment centers to health codes that permit involuntary detention and forced treatment to laws that allow for court-ordered treatment in the community. Although the laws, regulations, and policies described are specific to California, to the extent that such mechanisms exist in many other states and countries, we hope to furnish insights into how such euphemistically named concepts as assisted outpatient treatment function.

In Chapter 7, we begin by considering the effects of biopsychiatric power on individuals and in relation to the problem of homelessness. These considerations bring into sharp relief the extent to which the present system of mental health treatment is not only failing homeless citizens but increasing the potential for women to suffer further. In the second half of this chapter, we explore what an alternative mental health care system could look like and the benefits it could provide to individuals, families, communities, and the larger society.

Social Problems: A Final Consideration

As we previously stated, our primary interest in this book is in how biopsychiatric power manifests at the level of the individual and what the effects are for that individual. In placing the focus here, we are mindful of the fact that the problems of the people represented—homelessness, interpersonal violence, addiction, and mental health issues, among others—have social causes, meanings, and consequences. Although biopsychiatric power may be felt by particular individuals, it manifests through the institutions within which they are embedded. Thus, any attempt at hiving one off from other is inevitably doomed to fail at providing a fuller picture of the social phenomenon we are attempting to analyze.

Focusing exclusively on the micro level is an analytical strategy that carries with it other risks. As other commentators have noted (Lovell 1992; McKenzie-Mohr, Coates, and McLeod 2012), the medicalization and psychiatrization of homelessness has permitted a means for the social problems referenced above, principally homelessness, to be redefined, thus shifting the burden of responsibility away from policymakers and institutions onto the backs of those least able to defend themselves from misattribution and blame. Rendering social problems into forms of individual pathology also allows for maintenance of an unacceptable status quo, a point well captured by Ann Lovell:

> Using psychiatric status as an indicator of need presents a further danger. It promotes a circularity by which the supply defines the demand. That is, by defining the needs of homeless persons in terms of psychiatric dimensions and symptoms, the service itself—hospitalization or treatment—becomes the social goal. This circularity in turn legitimates and reinforces the existing system (or nonsystem) of services while preempting the possibility of other types of responses. It also removes from the universe of discourse (social policy) any indication of the macro-level changes that create and affect the day-to-day situation of homeless persons. It also removes from the universe of discourse (social policy) any indication of the macro-level changes that create and affect the day-today situation of homeless persons. (1992, p. 256)

A goal in this book is to use the same analytical strategy to invert the logic underlying the politics of biopsychiatry and to do so by using women's stories to reveal how the act of pathologizing individuals, and then inadequately treating their ascribed pathology, does little to solve the problems biopsychiatry purports to address. Indeed, more often than not, the acts of defining, treating, and enforcing compliance simply perpetuate or exacerbate these problems. That said, we return to our earlier contention that providing a fuller account of a given phenomenon, or a solution to a particular social problem, is impossible when individuals are treated as discrete entities that function separately from institutions, social structures, and processes. Thus, where appropriate, we will shift from a focus on the individual to the institutional, from the institutional to the social, and vice versa. Despite such attempts at providing what we hope to be simultaneously a broader and more detailed account, we are deeply cognizant of the fact that there is always so much more to be said.

Notes

1. Throughout this book the nonproprietary (generic) name is used in reference to or when discussing a particular psychiatric drug. However, when quoting a participant or another author or trying to clarify something for the reader, the appropriate brand name is left or added where referenced.

2. We employ the term *biopsychiatry* here to refer specifically to this branch of the general field of psychiatry. Although it is the predominant worldview found within contemporary psychiatry, as well as an influence on the work of practitioners in allied fields, it is not the only form of psychiatry presently in existence. Others include social psychiatry and cross-cultural psychiatry. Thus, we use *psychiatry* to refer to the field as a whole and *biopsychiatry* when discussing that body of research and clinical practice predicated on the belief that manifestations of human suffering are forms of mental illness largely, if not wholly, with biomedical causes.

3. Such medical practices were rooted in the ancient Greek humoral theory that tied disease to a variety of diverse imbalances, including those of the four humors (blood, phlegm, black bile, and yellow bile), four bodily conditions (hot, cold, wet, and dry), and the four corresponding elements (earth, air, fire, and water). Physicians were to balance these humors though treatments that were "opposite" to the symptoms. For example, bloodletting was a treatment to remove what was believed to be excess blood when a patient was flush due to being fevered (i.e., hot) (Kaufman 1988). This notion of allopathy has, although with contention, been applied to Western medicine to refer to a reliance on pharmaceutical and surgical treatments.

4. Prescription privileges vary by state. In California, registered nurses and pharmacists are permitted to prescribe drugs.

5. Again, our focus in this book—what we take issue with—is when such drugs are prescribed without being accompanied by any counseling, treatment, or trauma-informed care.

6. For example, dire outcomes, including suicidal ideations and feelings, were tied to the use of Paxil, especially among youths (Campbell 2010; Sexton 2003).

7. Ben-Moshe, Chapman, and Carey (2014) draw attention to falsities in historical understandings in explaining how the belief that the deinstitutionalization of people in treatment centers resulted in increased prison populations is not supported by demographic information. Instead they show how the prison boom accompanying deinstitutionalization was male and nonwhite rather than paralleling the demographic composition of the deinstitutionalized population. In this context, many of the victims of deinstitutionalization likely ended up on the streets.

8. Seventy-seven ($n = 77$) of those interviews were personally conducted by Laura Huey, and at least half a dozen of the remaining number were conducted under her direct supervision. An important point: although many of the participants in this study had been diagnosed with a mental illness, usually depression or an anxiety disorder, a principal requirement of study participation was the ability to give informed consent. Thus, if any woman appeared to be incapable of giving that consent (i.e., seemed intoxicated or exhibited signs to suggest that she was actively delusional at that time), we skipped the interview, and she was given a gift card and thanked for her time.

9. Although we do not make use of those earlier interviews in Detroit, Chicago, Liverpool, and Manchester in this book, we may include Huey's experiences in these sites when illustrating a salient point.

2

Empowered or Powerless?

Ellen is a forty-five-year-old African American woman who has been residing in a shelter since she lost her apartment. Her story is simple: she was let go from her job when she developed anxiety and depression following several workplace-related incidents. As she explains, "I knew something was wrong when I couldn't go to work. I was dressed, in uniform, ready to walk out the door, and just couldn't do it." Feeling helpless, she used her company-sponsored insurance to access mental health treatment. Of the process, she says:

> It started off as talk therapy. Then they asked me if I wanted to see the other doctor about some medication. I just wanted to talk to find out what the problem was. They told me they may never figure out what the problem is. I guess they were being truthful. After a couple months, nothing was improving, and everything was getting worse, so I said that I would take the pills.

Having lost her job, her home, the insurance to pay for continuing treatment, and the sense that she might "figure out what the problem is" underlying her anxiety and depression, Ellen has a new solution: "I was thinking about going into the hospital to straighten it out. Take all of my vitamins. Take all of the pill samples. Take all of the tests. I thought about taking two pinks and a yellow, and then I would be fine."

In Ellen's case, the "yellow" and the "pink" pills bring temporary relief to her symptoms of anxiety by dampening the thoughts and feelings that threaten to overwhelm her—that is, through sedation. As a result, and despite the fact Ellen is no closer to finding a cure for her condition, she is convinced that the solution to her problems lies in having medical doctors submit her to a battery of diagnostic tests, from which they will determine the best cocktail of psychiatric drugs to treat her condition. What makes this situation somewhat concerning is that in unpacking her story, one can see that the cause of her distress is obviously not unknown, that what she is experiencing are the effects of trauma. Despite the clear association, Ellen, like many other women, has never been exposed to trauma-informed therapeutic work or to any of the forms of psychotherapy that have proven to have some success in treating anxiety and depression.[1] Instead, what might properly be considered a failure of the mental health system to provide appropriate therapy has been transformed through the acts of diagnosis and prescription into a biochemical malfunction within Ellen's brain. This conclusion is not to suggest that anything inherent to trauma-informed care would preclude the use of psychotropic medication; rather, we are quite simply suggesting such medication may be more successful when accompanied by trauma-informed care.

A reader might be forgiven for thinking that Ellen's experience is somehow unique to her and to other impoverished women, easily explained as the result of a lack of access to quality medical care. It is not. It is a consequence of how the mental health field more generally, as well as a wide swath of society, views mental health.

The controversies over the DSM across history stem, in part, from the different classifications processes and views of mental health that have been used to determine what is included, why, and how the included conditions are organized in the manual. For example, the DSM-I, published in 1952 by the Committee on Nomenclature and Statistics of the American Psychiatric Association (APA), focused on clinical diagnoses and reflected Adolf Meyer's psychobiological perspective (i.e., mental disorders are maladaptive personality "reactions" to socioenvironmental, social, psychological, and biological factors) by using the word *reaction* throughout (APA 2015; Pressman 1997). Later, the DSM-II (1968) removed the term *reaction* yet was otherwise rather similar to the DSM-I (Wilson and Spitzer 1968). The DSM-III (1980) marked a paradigm shift in psychiatry by including more specific diagnostic criteria, among other changes based largely on empirical work (Kawa and Giordano 2012). This version was later revised (DSM-III-R in 1987) in light of inconsistencies and unclear diagnostic criteria. The DSM-IV (1994) added, deleted, and reorganized the disorders, changing the classifications, diagnostic criteria, and information provided in light of literature reviews and research (Kawa and Giordano 2012). It was followed by the DSM-IV-TR (text revised), which acknowledged cultural variability in how "mental health and illness are expressed and construed" (Kawa and Giordano 2012, p. xx).

Lloyd Rogler's (1997) analysis of the DSM further drew attention to the dominance of the medical model in its reiterations since DSM-III. Consistent with Rogler's work, controversies tied to the release of the DSM-V (2013) are most pertinent to our study of homeless women in Los Angeles, specifically the continued attempt to make the DSM rather pathophysiological or biological in nature when little evidence has been found of specific biological markers of mental illness. Even prior to the DSM-V's release, Shadia Kawa and James Giordano noted:

> Of particular interest is the continuing emphasis on the (at least implicit) incorporation of biological data into the classification of disorders in the DSM, with the intended elaboration of findings from studies in behavioural genetics and neuroimaging in the disorder classifications in the DSM-V. However, the Manual does not explicitly specify what and how neurogentic, neuroimaging, and neurochemical data can or should be employed in establishing differential diagnoses of mental disorders. (2012, p. 6; see Giordano 2012 for additional information)

Further, they explain that one of the most notable outcomes of the "symptom-based, somatically oriented descriptive approach fostered by the DSM-III is the *increase* in psychopharmacological interventions, applied to conditions ranging from the severest of mental disorders to much milder DSM categories *that had previously been treated with psychotherapeutic and behavioural approaches*" (Kawa and Giordano 2012, p. 7; emphasis added). Although some conditions, as a result, have been successfully treated with such drugs, this pharmacological approach has poor outcomes for many and can easily be tied to misuse (Healy 2004; Lane 2006).

Further, over the past few decades, individuals living in the West have been on the receiving end of a constant barrage of media citing studies and expert opinion declaring that depression and other mental health conditions are diseases caused by chemical imbalances in the brain. Less frequently discussed, if ever, is that this hypothesis—for that is what it is—has been supported by often dubious research sponsored by pharmaceutical companies (Healy 2012). In this sense, a criticism consistent with that awarded to the medical or allopathic models, the DSM in its more recent reiterations appears to depend on standardized testing and criteria with minimal regard for socioenvironmental and personal factors, including the impact such factors may have on the presentation of symptoms of conditions in people who may or may not benefit from treatment. Indeed, homeless women will easily present with symptoms of distress, meeting, like most in the United States, diagnostic criteria of some mental health conditions. They are in distress because, among other factors, they have no home!

Either way, the hypothesis that mental illnesses are the result of chemical imbalances in the brain has been contradicted by other studies that highlight a more complex nonbiological reality: symptoms of mental illness are frequently found to be distinct responses to trauma and other significant stressors in the lives of those diagnosed with mental disorders (Bentall 2009; Hammersley et al. 2003).

Within this chapter we provide an overview of sorts to help contextualize the material that follows. We begin with a discussion of Skid Row in Los Angeles as seen in light of structural violence. We use structural violence here to reveal the nuances underlying and beyond the system-wide gaps in dealing with homelessness before we focus on biopsychiatry. Next we explore the multifaceted stigma engulfing homeless women and how it reinforces power relations, including the powers of medicalization and psychiatrization. We then draw attention to the medical and biopsych model of mental health and how it has come to dominate not only the field of psychiatry but the way those in the West increasingly think about and respond to both individual and social problems. Then we look more closely at the role of biopsychiatry in the treatment of homelessness as a social problem, examining, in particular, what the relevant literature has had to say about how the three manifestations of psychiatric power—the powers to diagnose, prescribe, and garner compliance—affect the lives of homeless women. Lastly, we conclude by offering an alternative lens through which to view much of what has been understood as mental illness within homeless populations, a lens that focuses attention on the role of trauma in creating the signs of distress so frequently interpreted as symptoms of a disease.

Structural Violence

As a space, Skid Row exposes its inhabitants to experiences of both visible and direct *and* invisible and indirect violence. The latter form of violence, frequently termed *structural violence*, permeates the lives of homeless women. Structural violence is embedded within political and economic realities, and the experience of it is shaped by gender, race, geography, and socioeconomic factors (Bourgois, Prince, and Moss 2004; Farmer 2004, 2009; Hodgetts et al. 2014; Kelly 2005; Smith 2015; Zizek 2008). We use the term here because this use allows for implicit recognition of the fact that some individuals' lives are marked by experiences of significant institutional and economic hardships because of their relative status in life, a fact that is normalized in society (Bourgois, Prince, and Moss 2004; Zizek

2008). As Slovaj Zizek (2008) suggests, structural violence tends to be invisible because those most affected by it are marginalized by geography, class, race, or culture (see also Farmer 2009). Further, any suffering that results can be neither measured by observers nor conveyed to those who are not directly experiencing it. To illustrate, we note that homeless populations are generally spatially segregated (in our study reside on Skid Row) and often removed from the resources and programs required to meet their basic needs.

Due to the fact that the status of women is almost always inferior to that of men, gender-based power differentials in society, like poverty, systemically leave women more susceptible to physical and sexual violence (Farmer 2009). The social conditions that embody structural violence are not necessary violent, but the disproportionate and negative impact from them on specific social groups, like women, is a form of violence (Hodgetts et al. 2014). They are most often affected by indirectly exerted violence imposed through conditions outside their control, such as policies, legislation, and social interactions (see Bourgois, Prince, and Moss 2004; Farmer 2004, 2009; Hodgetts et al. 2014; Zizek 2008). Structural violence then restricts the agency and limits access to resources, such as food and medicine, of its victims, who often do not know how to cope with said realities (Farmer 2004). Philippe Bourgois and his colleagues (2004) argue, for example, that interpersonal violence in poor neighborhoods often stems from frustrations and blocked lives tied to structural violence, producing a violent backdrop to the seeming peace that permeates everyday life in the absence of interpersonal violence.

Political Ideologies

Structured violence is linked to the capitalist desire for profit, which creates indifference toward the structured inequities among citizens (Zizek 2008). Under the umbrella of the US form of neoliberal capitalism, political ideology reproduces power relationships that are detrimental for those in the lower social-economic tiers, yet the perpetrators of violence are not tangible or fixed (Zizek 2008). Those who impose the practices and policies that regulate and control individual behavior are not directly affected by the policies themselves. For example, in a study of the interactions between government workers and 100 families who accessed food banks on a regular basis in Auckland, New Zealand, Darrin Hodgetts and colleagues (2014) reveal the structural violence underlying the limited access to resources, volatile and hostile social interactions, and harsh and dehumanizing landscapes imposed on those seeking services. They point out how these forms of violence result from political ideologies, not the workers themselves, and how policymakers often fail to experience the negative and sometimes harsh consequences of their actions. Political ideologies then, in addition to stigmatized views of specific social groups, continue this form of violence in social experiences (e.g., face-to-face interactions, landscapes) and symbolic spaces through representational politics (e.g., policy documents, media reports) (Zizek 2008).

Turning to a more relevant example, in North America, Brendan Kelly (2005) examines the structural violence experienced by individuals living with schizophrenia and its impact on their health (e.g., disease onset, diagnosis, treatment options). He demonstrates how political factors manifest in the clinical and social features of the disorder, worsening the individual's health condition. For instance, although schizophrenia is historically seen as a biological illness, it continues to have a disproportionate impact on homeless and migrant populations, who are more likely to experience earlier onset and delayed diagnosis:

> The adverse effects of these social, economic, and societal factors, along with the social stigma of mental illness, constitute a form of "structural violence" which impairs access to psychiatric and social services and amplifies the effects of schizophrenia in the lives of sufferers. As a result of these over-arching social and economic factors, many individuals with schizophrenia are systematically excluded from full participation in civic and social life, and are constrained to live lives that are shaped by stigma, isolation, homelessness and denial of rights. (Kelly 2005, p. 721)

In this context, clearly the practices and systems put in place indirectly, and at times unintentionally, inflict violence on vulnerable social groups by creating a system in which they must struggle to survive (Hodgetts et al. 2014). Further, this violence places them in an inferior position, unable to advocate for their own healthcare needs or even to resist the pressures to adhere to the directives of medical professionals. This situation is not surprising given the stigma tied to most mental disorders, particularly the delusional disorders such as schizophrenia.

Stigma

Literally defined as a "mark of infamy" or "brand" (Sadow and Ryder 2008), stigma imposes a "marked identity" outside the realm of what is culturally read as normal on a person (Phelan and Link 2004, 2011). This process often includes making stigmatized people's virtual social identities salient and discrediting their actual social identities (Goffman 1963). The former includes attributes or qualities "marked" individuals are thought to possess where the latter is the identity they do possess. Said another way, the actual social identity is disregarded, and the individual becomes identified by the stigmatizing attribute (Goffman 1963). Stigmatizing individuals with undesirable labels ensures that they become viewed as inferior persons, the stigma "reduc[ing] the bearer from a whole and usual person to a tainted, discounted one" (Goffman 1963, p. 3). Although stigma has many facets, it is often indicative of structural violence: for example, the mental health stigma is the result of dynamic processes where one is branded within a social context (see Dalky 2012).

As with mental illness, Bourgois and his colleagues (2004) explain that individuals existing in what is culturally read as the "lower social tiers of society" bear the stigma of their social, economic, and political position and are thus negatively viewed, which in turn manifests into forms of violence. Beyond the too common outcome of victim blaming, the lived experiences of marginalized and vulnerable populations become seen as a consequence of self-destructive behaviors, and any social or economic factors determining their realities are ignored and forgotten (Bourgois, Prince, and Moss 2004). In a study of homeless women in San Francisco struggling with heroin addiction and thus susceptible to hepatitis C, for example, Bourgois and colleagues (2004) found that even people tasked with helping these women associated their risk-taking behaviors, like sharing needles, water, and cookers, to the negative attributes they were believed to possess. Specifically, they were thought to be ignorant, psychopathic, and immoral. The stigma these women bore was further reflected in many of the policies and practices put in place to supply what authorities saw as help, policies that resulted in the women's further marginalization. For instance, in promoting messages about how to minimize risk-taking behaviors, health professionals ignored the intimate relationships these women had with their partners, partners who too often only allow women to use heroin with them. Although a form of control that perpetuates further violence, many women saw this manipulation as a symbolic manifestation of their partners' love and commitment (Bourgois, Prince, and Moss 2004). Unfortunately, none of the messages oriented to keeping these women safe and healthy addressed such problems, which reflects larger relationships of power and social and economic constraints. In the case of these women, their risky behavior (e.g., exposure to hepatitis C) was a consequence of their addiction, relationships with their partners, and need for survival in their current environment, not a result of a lack of care or concern for their health. The latter conclusion evidences structural violence and the assumptions made about these women—stereotypes and stigma—that have an impact on their life choices and limit available supports or resources (Bourgois, Prince, and Moss 2004).

Of course, one cannot ignore how structural violence underpins instances where people who fail to sustain themselves and families or meet current standards of self-reliance are met with punitive responses (Hodgetts et al. 2014). Said another way, linking poverty to individual shortcomings rather than economic, social, or environmental factors reveals the stigma imposed upon individuals and the structural violence embedded in social systems and institutions (Hodgetts et al. 2014). People living in poverty are stigmatized, yet in blaming them for their own positioning, structural violence is justifiable; thus the poorer treatment of groups of individuals and the minimal support provided to them can be condoned by the government (Hodgetts et al. 2014).

Medicalization

The process of medicalization is shaped by both stigma and structural violence. We are hardly alone in this insight. Medical anthropologists have long recognized the role and cumulated effects of structural violence, discrimination, and stigma in generating the suffering that then is thought to require biomedical, including biopsychological, intervention (e.g., Baer, Singer, and Susser 1997; Kim et al. 2000; Rylko-Bauer and Farmer 2002). At the conceptual level, medicalization occurs when symptoms with what is in essence a social origin, like stresses and anxieties, are labeled in medical jargon and deemed to require medical intervention if the individual is to recover. Stress, including what some medical anthropologists have labeled *oppression illness* (Baer, Singer, and Susser 1997), is treated as a mental illness requiring intervention once medicalized. Oppression illness, however, in actuality is "a product of the impact of suffering from social mistreatment . . . and, at some level, accepting blame for one's suffering as just retribution for someone who does not deserve better treatment. . . . The source of stress is being the object of widespread and enduring social discrimination, degradation, structural violence and abusive derision" (Singer 2004, p. 17). Thus, the medicalization of the outcomes of oppressive social relationships and environments reflects how the positions of marginalized and vulnerable populations remain unchanged. Indeed, as an illustration, Merrill Singer (2004) notes the irony that, although drug addiction is a clinical disorder, drug users are incarcerated for petty crimes instead of sent for treatment. This situation in effect reinforces and maintains the addict's marginalized and vulnerable position in society. In a similar vein, although focused on political violence and ethnic conflict, Duncan Pedersen argues that "the medicalization of collective suffering and trauma reflects a poor understanding of the relationships among critically important social determinants and the range of possible health outcomes" (2002, p. 175). He could easily have been speaking about homelessness and other such realities.

Medicalization also occurs at the interactional level. It is evinced in the social interactions between those in need of assistance, in our study homeless women, and the service providers, including medical professionals, from whom they seek help or treatment. Practitioners serve as the gatekeepers to said help. They have access to needed resources and services yet potentially, though often unintentionally, reinforce in their practices elements of the violent systems and ideologies structuring society. Akhil Gupta (2013) demonstrates how, in the delivery of welfare services, providers by appearing callous and not empathetic can impose violent conditions on those seeking access to these services. Further, choosing to limit—despite how this decision is justified—access can further marginalize those with the greatest need. Bringing Gupta's work back to the medicalization of trauma and homelessness, the actions of professionals who are often simply following institutional guidelines may have a negative impact on already vulnerable populations, reinforce stigma, and further hinder access to basic services and resources. Indeed, the treatment of the symptoms of patients' mental disorders is where existing power relations between social groups can be reproduced and maintained: the service providers or doctors have power, and the patients' well-being is tended to in accordance with their discretions. Further the practitioners' actions are shaped by the policies, practices, stigma, and values underlying institutional structures, which also affect their demeanor and interactions with "clients." This influence was empirically documented in Hodgetts and colleagues' (2014) study of interactions between individuals' living in urban poverty and service providers or government workers. What this study reveals is how such interactions are often laced with judgments, a lack of sympathy, hostility, and a callous demeanor toward those seeking assistance (Hodgetts et al. 2014). Thus, structural violence and stigma shape medicalized realities at the conceptual, interactional, and institutional levels, something that became increasing evident in the positioning of biopsychiatry as an institution.

Within the scope of biopsychiatry, at the institutional level, medical personnel supervise treatment, act as gatekeepers to treatment or care, and determine when lived experiences become redefined as illness requiring intervention (Armstrong and Armstrong 2010). Recognizing that, at each level, relationships of power frame the experiences of those seeking aid, we now turn to unpacking the history of biopsychiatry as an institution with governance over "sick people." In doing so, we see how violence can be institutionalized and indirectly structure practices that fall under the realm of biopsychiatry.

A Worldview

Although many commentators set the beginnings of biopsych in the 1950s with the discovery of the major tranquilizers (neuroleptics), evidence of the workings of an organic model in psychiatric practice is seen in earlier treatments oriented toward identifying, removing, and treating pathological functioning within the body (Tasca et al. 2012).[2] And certainly the use of psychoactive drugs to treat defined psychiatric conditions was not new either: for instance, from the 1930s on, amphetamines were administered to those diagnosed with depression and manic depression, today more commonly known as bipolar disorders I and II.[3] Regardless of this fact, the discovery of the neuroleptic chlorpromazine, an antipsychotic, antiemetic drug, is more often credited with engendering an era of renewed interest in biopsychiatry (c.f. Breggin 1991). What makes the story somewhat ironic is that chlorpromazine was created in 1951 as a general anesthetic for surgery and not for a psychiatric purpose (Ban 2007). Its potential use as a tranquilizer to sedate psychiatric patients was discovered accidentally when a French army surgeon, Henri Laborit, began studying chlorpromazine as a means of preventing surgical shock (Ban 2007). Noting that chlorpromazine produced a disinterested effect on patients, he persuaded doctors at the Val-de-Grâce military hospital in Paris to use chlorpromazine to treat one of their psychotic patients (Ban 2007). Given that it was intended to anesthetize surgical patients, the drug not surprisingly produced an immediate calming effect (Ban 2007). Subsequent clinical investigations confirmed that chlorpromazine could be used to control the behaviors of manic patients (Bentall 2009). Its introduction for clinical use was shortly followed by the release of the first prescribed psychoactive drug to make a larger cultural impact: meprobamate, marketed as Miltown (Marshall, Georgievskava, and Georgievsky 2009). Miltown, which had a mild sedative effect on patients, was released in 1955 for the treatment of anxiety, thus becoming the first of the "minor tranquilizers" (Marshall, Georgievskava, and Georgievsky 2009). It was followed by the introduction of the benzodiazepines (i.e., Librium and Valium) (Marshall, Georgievskava, and Georgievsky).

In retrospect, cultural shifts often read as inexorable, inevitable processes; however, there was nothing inexorable or inevitable about the rise of biopsych and the worldview it espouses. Instead, one can see an enacted power to further stigmatize a vulnerable population and an "other" people in need of help who struggle with their personal and cognitive well-being, another example of structural violence. Biopsych, in essence, confirms that something is wrong that needs fixing, which then reinforces the authority of medical practitioners and the structure of the allopathic medical model. The emphasis on chemical treatments simply flourishes alongside, not coincidentally, the economic governance of the pharmaceutical industry, as will be discussed.

As such with the discovery of their ability to alter behavior through the administration of psychoactive drugs, a cadre of psychiatric researchers and clinicians began to push for wider acceptance of a biomedical model of cognitive and behavioral functioning rooted in the idea that mental health problems were manifestations of underlying disorders with biological causes, not at all unlike the diseases studied by other medical disciplines (Moncrieff 2013). Over the course of the 1960s and 1970s, such views began to gain ground within the psychiatric community because of a set of factors that were vital to the field's growth.

First, recognition of the limitations of the psychoanalytic model and the failure of the psy sciences to successfully produce alternative explanatory models was growing (Bentall 2009). As human nature abhors a vacuum, the resulting gap was readily filled by the new paradigm, actively promoted by a number of prominent biopsych proponents who gained increasing influence within the discipline (Aho 2008). Indeed, how much their efforts paid off is evident in the publication of the DSM-III (1984), which firmly propelled psychiatry toward a more biopsychiatric orientation by purging psychoanalytical concepts from the manual (Frances 2013). To illustrate, relatively amorphous psychoanalytical constructs such as neurosis were replaced with anxiety disorders, mood disorders, and dissociative disorders, each tied to a specific symptomology that supposedly could be observed, measured, and thus standardized (Frances 2013). Much was riding on this change: as Joanna Moncrieff suggests, "the credibility of the modern DSM and similar systems . . . lies in the implication that the various labels they propose indicate the presence of an underlying disease, which particular treatments can target and rectify . . . [and] if the process of diagnosis cannot direct the choice of treatment, then it has no practical or convincing purpose" (2013, p. 214). The result of these changes, she notes, is that psychiatric theory has become "a self-perpetuating cycle, with the illness model of mental disturbance justified by the disease-centred model of drug action, which was itself bolstered by the idea that mental disorders are properly thought of as discrete, biologically-based diseases" (p. 214).

Second, as an interdisciplinary enterprise, biopsych aligns psychiatry with neuroscience, biochemistry, genetics, and psychopharmacology, producing a unified field of research. This alliance has the additional and not coincidental benefit of allowing the discipline of psychiatry to more firmly establish itself within the domain known as hard science and thus to confer greater professional prestige on its practitioners. No longer tied to such professionally problematic creatures as Sigmund Freud or Carl Jung, their work would now have the imprimatur of so-called real medicine. Illustrative of this ambition were the remarks of Robert Spitzer, the APA chair of the group tasked with revising the DSM-III, who opined that his group's adoption of the biopsych approach within the discipline's diagnostic bible signaled an "achievement for psychiatry" because it represented "an advancement toward the fulfillment of the scientific aspirations of the profession" (Bayer and Spitzer 1985, p. 187).

Third, as is now known, research and education on the question of how to regulate what those in the field thought of as biological dysfunction—the brain's chemical imbalances—was supported by generous funding from pharmaceutical companies (Frances 2013; Kutchins and Kirk 1997). The pharmaceutical industry's contribution, as we previously noted, to the rise of biopsych is at least twofold, both laced with evidence of structural violence and the increasing medicalization of conditions of being. First, pharmaceutical companies sponsored research aimed at proffering support for the chemical imbalance hypothesis and demonstrating the efficacy of their drugs for the treatment of these purported imbalances. How much of the pharma-related research presented in journals and at conferences is in fact either drawn from researchers' analyses of the raw data produced in pharma-sponsored clinical trials or is even written by the researchers themselves is debatable. David Healy (2012), who has written on the practice of the ghost-writing of research papers, suggests that a portion of the research in this area is not the work of independent scientists but rather industry spin disguised as scientific data (see also Sismondo 2007).

The second means by which the pharmaceutical industry has promoted biopsych is through spending vast sums on "educating" psychiatrists, the scientific community, and the public on the benefits of "better living through chemistry" (Bentall 2009; Frances 2013). One of the major beneficiaries of the pharmaceutical industry's largesse has been the APA, which received revenues from pharmaceutical advertising, sponsored "education" programs, and research subsidies and sponsorship of its annual meetings (APA 2010). In 2006 alone the APA received over $18 million in financial support from pharmaceutical companies (APA 2010). Over time, evidence of widespread industry funding and its real and perceived effects on research, clinical work, and education began to prompt a backlash within the psychiatric community, with several prominent figures speaking publicly about what they saw as the co-opting of their discipline (notably, Angell 2000 and Frances 2013). Faced with a public relations disaster, the APA decided to act in 2009 by limiting its dependence on industry funding. By 2012, funding of APA activities by pharmaceutical companies was down to $5.6 million; however, this funding remains a considerable source of financial support for the association (APA 2012).

In looking at the rise of biopsych, one must also consider the cultural element. Buoyed in part by the success in the 1970s of diazepam (Valium, which slows the nerves in the central nervous system and thus has a calming effect), by the late 1980s biopsych was arguably well on its way to becoming not only a cultural force but the zeitgeist of a set of increasingly anxious and depressed populations. What undoubtedly helped push it into becoming *the* dominant frame through which much of these populations came to understand mental health issues and, increasingly, ordinary woes was the introduction of the second generation of antidepressants. Of these, the most notable for its cultural impact is fluoxetine (more commonly known as Prozac, a selective serotonin reuptake inhibitor [SSRI] antidepressant used to treat depression, among other conditions). The success of fluoxetine was astounding. First introduced onto the market in 1988, within two years over 10 million prescriptions for its use had been generated, with that number doubling by 1996 (Marshall, Georgievskava, and Georgievsky 2009). What makes fluoxetine's early success particularly remarkable is that its manufacturer, Eli Lilly, did not begin direct-to-consumer advertising of this product until 1996 (Marshall et al. 2009), thus early prescription rates cannot be attributed to direct appeals to consumers through sad-faced images on their television screens. This point is made not to say that fluoxetine was not featured in mass media products; indeed, a caption proclaiming it as "a breakthrough drug for depression" could be found on the cover of a 1990 issue of *Newsweek*, complete with a story extolling the perceived virtues of its use (Marshall, Georgievskava, and Georgievsky 2009). News and television articles were joined by a raft of books. Among these were the best sellers *Listening to Prozac*, by the psychiatrist Peter Kramer (1993), and Elizabeth Wurtzel's (1994) memoir, *Prozac Nation*. By 2000, the name *Prozac* had become such a staple of popular culture that the name could be found within the dictionary of a popular word processing program (Freemantle and Mason 2000). Since 2007 the US Food and Drug Administration (FDA) has required the makers of antidepressants (including Eli Lilly for Prozac) to update the "black-box" warning—the most aggressive precaution available for any drug, which must appear on its label to call attention to serious or life-threatening risks—about the risk of suicidal ideations and behavior during early treatment (Friedman 2014). This requirement is telling given the black-box warning is the strongest precaution the FDA can issue other than recalling and no longer allowing the drug to be sold on the market. Nonetheless, writing in 2015, although Prozac remains popular in use, it has been challenged by a host of other antidepressants that are demonstrating the enduring popularity of neurochemical solutions to the problems of modern cultures.

In order for biopsych to become the predominant lens through which issues of mental health are viewed, its central tenets had to be supported by another key group: clinicians. Unfortunately, little research has examined the influence of biopsych on practitioner practices. One notable exception is a series of studies conducted by a team of Yale researchers (Ahn, Proctor, and Flanagan 2009). In the first of these studies, a sample of registered psychiatrists, psychologists, social workers, psychiatry residents, psychology interns, and social work fellows were asked to attribute biological, psychological, or environmental causes to 445 mental disorders in order to determine how clinicians attributed causes to different disorders. The results indicate that, although the range of disorders was categorized as belonging to causes across the three domains, when a disorder was judged to be strongly biological in nature, it was deemed weakly psychological or environmental and vice versa. In other words, clinicians saw very little ambiguity when ascribing the causes and effects of disorders. Of particular interest is how a professional background had a significant effect on the degree experts judged whether a disorder was biological in cause: psychiatrists were most likely to ascribe a biological basis to a disorder, followed by psychologists and then social workers (Ahn, Proctor, and Flanagan 2009). To test the reliability of these results, the research team then selected nine disorders used in the first study (three viewed as most likely to be biological in nature, three deemed moderately biological, and three least likely to be biological) and asked a subset of participants to rate each according to whether it was seen as biological, psychological, or environmental in cause. The findings confirmed their previous results (Ahn, Proctor, and Flanagan 2009). It is, however, the third study that is particularly instructive in understanding the link between causal beliefs and prescribing practices. In this study, researchers presented a series of case histories to participants and asked them to judge the degree to which they believed psychiatric drugs or psychotherapy would be more useful for treating the pseudopatient. The results revealed that clinicians view psychiatric drugs as more effective in treating cases with attributed biological causes and therapy as more appropriate for cases involving social or environmental causes. Interestingly, the researchers note that "this was true even though both cases may be of the same disorder" (Ahn, Proctor, and Flanagan 2009, p. 164).

Another, albeit indirect, indicator of the extent to which clinicians tend to see mental health issues as being rooted in biological causes can be found in their willingness to prescribe drugs that would reverse the biochemical conditions they saw as creating the symptoms catalogued. Data from the United States on prescription patterns from two different sources paints a fairly startling picture. Figures extracted from a 2008 survey by the National Center for Health Statistics of the US Centers for Disease Control and Prevention reveal that antidepressants are among the top three drug classes most frequently prescribed for both teens and adults (Gu, Dillon, and Burt 2010). They are the top form of prescribed drug for adults (10.8 percent), beating out both analgesics (10.1 percent) and drugs for lowering cholesterol (8.4 percent) (Gu, Dillon, and Burt 2010). Figures released by IMS Institute for Healthcare Informatics (2014) from the National Prescription Audit reveal that an antianxiety drug and two forms of antidepressants (respectively) were among the top twenty-five drug prescriptions filled in the United States in 2013.

Economic incentives clearly underlie processes of medicalization. The trend toward prescription drug use as acceptable and useful treatments for an ever-increasing number of states of being, each medicalized under the umbrella of illness, reveals the authority and power awarded to practitioners in particular and the field of biopsychiatry more generally. Medicalizing unhappiness and eroding any perception that individuals can recover without depending on drugs to fix their purported chemical imbalance benefits pharmaceutical companies and makes the need for treatment providers, like psychiatrists, undisputable. Biopsychiatry occupies an empowered position, includes a range of psychiatric technologies, and in its practice perpetuates the stigmatization and subordination of vulnerable and marginalized populations.

Table 2.1 US Psychiatric Drug Spending in Relation to the Top 25 Dispensed (millions)

Dispensed Prescriptions	2008	2009	2010	2011	2012	2013
#13 alprazolam[a]	43.3	45.3	47.7	49.1	49.2	49.6
#18 sertraline[b]	33.7	34.8	36.2	37.6	39.2	41.7
#19 citalopram[b]	22.6	27.3	32.2	37.8	38.9	39.5

Notes: a. A central nervous system depressant, used primarily to treat anxiety caused by depression, among other conditions.

b. SSRIs used to treat depression, anxiety, OCD, and other conditions.

Biopsychiatry in the Lives of Homeless Citizens

Homelessness has long been seen as an individual and social problem, even a recognized consequence of structural violence, but properly falling within the domain of psychiatry. Indeed, some scholars suggest that the field of psychiatry owes its early existence to the perceived need to house and treat impoverished citizens: "The birthplace of the specialty of psychiatry was in the asylum . . . which was created to divert patients from workhouses where the most disadvantaged and destitute people with mental illness were to be found" (Abdul-Hamid and Bhui 2014, p. 71). For centuries, those individuals deemed mentally unfit and lacking the means to enter private facilities were segregated within public institutions. This mass confinement began to give way in the 1950s, with the beginnings of a deinstitutionalization movement aimed at placing individuals in independent living situations within the community (Krieg 2001). In the United States, this movement was facilitated by several factors, including a series of court cases that required states to develop less restrictive alternatives to long-term institutionalization (Krieg 2001). It was also greatly aided by the belief that community-based care would be cost effective for governments (Lamb and Bachrach 2001), along with being more eminently viable as a result of the introduction of psychotropic drugs (Krieg 2001).

For some two decades, following the start of the deinstitutionalization movement, issues related to poverty and mental health generated little public attention. This lack of social awareness began to change in the 1980s, with the increasing social visibility of economically and socially disenfranchised victims of, first, a stagnant economy and then of a set of harsh economic and social policies known as Reaganomics.[4] As a result, the issue of homelessness emerged both as a significant social problem within the public consciousness and as one that was largely viewed as a biopsychiatric problem (Fuller Torrey 1988). Certainly, as individuals manifesting overt signs of distress became increasingly visible within the urban landscape, their presence was used as support for the belief that deinstitutionalization had turned loose thousands of "crazies" who refused to engage in treatment and were now homeless as a direct result (the subtext of much of this theorizing being that their presence was creating something of an urban blight that needed to be remedied) (Fuller Torrey 1988). However, what is often overlooked in histories of the rediscovery of homelessness is the extent to which the biopsychiatrization of the problem was a direct result of the role of squads of researchers,[5] who set off to explore the causes and conditions of this phenomena as though they had come upon new and unchartered territory. Although some of this work examined the structural economic and social conditions that gave rise to urban poverty, seeing them as vehicles of structural violence tainted by the political and stereotypical views tied to marginalized groups (see Bourgois 1998; Bourgois, Prince, and Moss 2004; Gupta 2013; Hodgetts et al. 2014; Zizek 2008), a great deal of it was focused on the individual, in particular, on those behaviors deemed to be signs of innate pathology. Indeed, from the 1980s onward, study after study provided rates of various clinical diagnoses, from substance abuse to depression to schizophrenia. In essence, what the researchers told the public was that approximately one-third of the homeless population meet the diagnostic criteria for one or more mental disorders (Jencks 1994; Koegel, Burnam, and Farr 1988). And, if one includes substance abuse disorders, the overall rate of clinical disorders among homeless citizens was suggested to be closer to 75 percent (Markowitz 2006, 2011).

To be fair, the emphasis on individual pathology as a casual explanation for homelessness within the research literature was hardly unique to the biosciences (psychiatry, general medicine, and nursing, among them); it was also found within and across the social sciences, from our own disciplines of sociology and criminology to the fields of psychology and social work. Given the extent to which researchers continue to find relatively high rates of mental disorders within homeless populations, biopsychiatry unsurprisingly colonized this state as though it were a new territory. It did so in a number of ways. One was to declare "the homeless mentally ill . . . one of the greatest problems of present-day society" and strike up an APA task force to determine how biopsychiatry could best address the problem (Lamb and Talbott 1986, p. 498). The APA also lent its experts to various public policy initiatives, and its practitioners allied themselves with collaborative mental health programs.[6] For example, psychiatrists were instrumental in the development of a New York–based program, Project HELP, which included outreach, transitional community care, and involuntary emergency treatment components.

Such efforts did not require much public convincing; the stigmas tied to mental disorders and homelessness together make sure people who fit the profile are left fully exposed and thus in a state of total vulnerability. The APA's task force in itself reveals the power and persistence of structural violence in much the same way as Kelly (2005) showed how the discrimination and inequality shaping the treatment of mental health issues also create structural violence. In his study, the stigmatization of people living with schizophrenia specifically resulted in their systemic exclusion from full participation in society. Indeed, their lives are shaped by stigma, isolation, and denial of rights, which in turn justify the violence they experience (Kelly 2005). The enduring stigma and social exclusion of mental illness, alongside social, economic, and political factors (i.e., it can shape an individual's social and economic circumstances) constitute forms of structural violence that limit treatment options and amplify the effects of the disorder. The violence many marginalized populations experience is, in essence, justified by the stigmatized view society holds of them and their behaviors, which works in conjunction with political and economic factors to reproduce violent structures. As such, the ease with which the APA task force applied the label of "mental illness" to homeless populations is not surprising, nor was the creation of a task force to determine how biopsychiatry could be used to address the so-called problem (Lamb and Talbott 1986). Retrospectively, that homelessness too would become a medicalized reality in need of treatment seems inevitable.

Thus far the focus has been on how rates of psychiatric diagnoses have been used to convince the public and policymakers alike that the problem, and thus the solution, to some 33 to 75 percent of homelessness is rooted in causes that lie within the domain of biopsychiatry, perhaps an easy feat given the multifaceted stigma tied to mental disorders and the state of homelessness. One must remember, though, that attributions of cause carry with them important, though unspoken, assumptions for how a defined issue is understood and responded to and thus are about so much more than the act of simply slotting people into taxonomical schemes. In relation to the matter of understanding the connections drawn between homelessness and mental health, biopsych proponents have been fairly careful to avoid directly attributing the problems of a majority of homeless citizens to malfunctioning processes within their brains. In most instances, this attribution is simply implied or buried under disease metaphors. Some instances can be found, however, where such connections are made explicit: in an article on mental health problems reported by homeless women, the sociologist Erika Laine Austin and her colleagues note that "homelessness is frequently co-incident with *organic mental illness*" (2008, p. 26; emphasis added). Among disorders included in the DSM that are attributed to pathological processes within individual brains are bipolar disorder (BPD), schizophrenia, and major depression (Austin, Anderson, and Gelberg 2008).

Given what is known of the relationship between causal beliefs and clinician treatment practices in the mental health field, a discussion of prescription practices in treating homeless citizens within the relevant research would be a reasonable find to expect. Yet, to date, few researchers have even casually discussed psychoactive prescription patterns within this population, and to our knowledge no one has examined the issue in extensive detail. Cobbling together material from various sources, it would appear that, although any particular insight into the volume of psychiatric drug prescriptions provided within homeless communities, or the extent to which they are actually filled and consumed, is rather limited (Barber 2009; Whitney and Glazier 2004). Discussing his work with homeless citizens in New York during the 1980s and 1990s, Charles Barber offers the following description of the types of psychiatric drugs he observed being prescribed:

> To quell their unruly moods and their troublesome delusions and hallucinations, my patients were taking all manner of psychiatric medications. Some of these medications had been around since the 1950s and 1960s—mood stabilizers like lithium, antipsychotics such as Haldol and Thorazine—while others, at the time, were brand-new, with strange and exotic names like Prozac, Paxil, and Zoloft. Each year over the course of the 1990s, new psychiatric medications were introduced and consumed *en masse* by my clients. Some of these new medications arrived with great fanfare and extremely high expectations. In particular, a class of agents called "atypical antipsychotics"—Risperdal, Clozaril, and Zyprexa are the best known—had been shown in early clinical studies to be far superior to the Haldols and the Thorazines. Overnight, it seemed, almost all patients were converted to these new drugs, as well as new-generation antidepressants and mood stabilizers. (2009, p. 7)

Barber's words show that variety in psychiatric drugs seemed to grow significantly, almost exponentially, over time. More recently, authors examining a prescription-dispensing program in Los Angeles's Skid Row District noted that the most common psychotropic drugs prescribed in this community were antidepressants followed by antipsychotics (Chung et al. 2012).

Although the literature in this area is sparse, some sources make reference to the issue of polypharmacy within homeless communities. As an example, in a study of homeless youth, many participants "were on numerous combinations of medications, including antipsychotics, antidepressants, and anticonvulsants" (Muir-Cochrane et al. 2006, p. 168). Similarly, Barber says, "It was not at all unusual for my clients to be taking three, four, five, or six different types of psychiatric drugs in a given day—a combination not unlike the number of street drugs many of them had once been addicted to" (2009, p. 7). Particularly concerning here is that many antidepressants, including SSRIs, have been found to increase suicidal thoughts and behaviors among youth (see Campbell 2010; Sexton 2003).

Thus far we have examined what the literature reveals about how the powers of definition and prescription manifest in the lives of homeless citizens, but what of the third power, the ability to garner compliance through interinstitutional alliances? Whereas the literature on prescribing patterns in homeless communities is thin, slightly more has been written on the issue of compliance, in particular, on the failure of homeless citizens to follow prescription drug treatments and the need to find mechanisms to enforce treatment. In relation to noncompliance, what is known, in essence, is that some homeless citizens refuse prescribed psychiatric drugs or cease taking them after a period of initial use. Among reasons for discontinuing treatment, homeless citizens cite mild to severe physical side effects, a fear of becoming dependent on prescribed drugs, and an inability to access, store, or keep their prescriptions safe from theft (Muir-Cochrane et al. 2006; Whitney and Glazier 2004). The literature on patient compliance reveals a continuum of control, ranging from soft (persuasion) to hard (physical coercion) forms of enforcement. At the softer end of the spectrum are programs variously termed *assertive community treatment* (Dixon et al. 1997) or *shelter-based collaborative mental health* (Stergiopoulos, Rouleau, and Yoder 2007), within which individuals are variously educated, inveigled, and bribed into complying with treatment. Depending on the perceived complexity of the issues presented, within such programs individuals are typically referred to either a primary care physician or psychiatrist for diagnosis and treatment (Stergiopoulos, Rouleau, and Yoder 2007). Treatment typically includes daily consumption of prescribed drugs or the administration of depot drugs, typically injectable long-acting antipsychotics (Stergiopolous, Rouleau, and Yoder 2007).

For those who are not amenable to adhering to prescribed treatment and who are deemed a risk to themselves or others, various jurisdictions, including Los Angeles, increasingly rely on mental health courts to enforce treatment. As with other specialized courts, mental health courts allow, as an alternative to incarceration, for the diversion of any person who has committed a criminal offense who has also been diagnosed with a mental disorder into community-based forms of treatment. Notably, a frequent precondition of diversion is the person's agreement to adhere to court-ordered mental health treatment, which typically entails compliance with a prescribed psychiatric drug regimen (Hughes and Peak 2013). Another mechanism for garnering drug treatment compliance is through the use of community treatment orders, a legal device found across the United States (including California) and in a number of other countries. Laws providing for community treatment orders typically come in one of four forms: as a form of conditional release from involuntary admission, as a diversion from compulsory inpatient treatment, as a preventive order for an individual deemed at risk who does not meet involuntary admission criteria, and as court-ordered treatment under guardianship laws (Snow and Austin 2009). As these scholars note, failure to observe mandated treatment, whether it be psychosocial or pharmaceutical in nature, can result in involuntary confinement and treatment (Snow and Austin 2009). Lastly, should someone be deemed as being at risk or as presenting a risk to others in the community, state health codes permit the arrest, detention, and involuntary treatment of individuals at inpatient psychiatric wards. Of course, both forced treatment and involuntary confinement are sometimes necessary for the well-being of the individual and can even be lifesaving interventions. And, in some instances, a diagnosis of a mental illness, substance abuse issues, or disability can in turn open up access to more services and resources. However, unfortunately, although homeless citizens have been subject to involuntary confinement and forced treatment, this phenomenon has generated little scholarly attention.

An Alternate Stating of the Problem

The contribution of biopsychiatry (or biopsych) to current psy science discourse is most recognized in its role in the creation of diagnostic classifications and criteria, the study of pharmacological effects of various psychiatric drugs on identified symptoms, and the generation of a substantial body of research aimed at identifying perceived biomechanical causes of mental disorders. Again, some of this research has been focused on proving the chemical deficiency hypothesis, whereas other research has been focused on anatomical structures or on attempts to identify candidate genes linked to specific emotional or behavioral abnormalities. Despite enormous efforts in these directions, though, to date the single most predictive factor associated with the mental disorders we explore in this book remains an environmental one: trauma, including trauma tied to structural violence in its diverse forms.

Before we begin, we should perhaps situate ourselves: regarding the nature-nurture divide, we are not, nor have ever been, purists. All behavior, cognition, and feeling are biological in the sense that they are products of a mind that is housed within a material entity: the brain. The development and functioning of that brain, as in all brains, is dependent on genetics. Until scientists discover the existence of a new emotion, we can assuredly say that in the normal, healthy brain, a circumscribed set of possibilities can be described with respect to individual temperaments and feelings. What makes each human being unique is that he or she is a product not only of genes but of the complex interplay between developmental, environmental, and social factors. Where we perhaps differ from biopsych proponents is in our insistence, as sociologists and criminologists, on foregrounding the social over the biological, particularly in insisting on the significance of traumatic experience in shaping thoughts, feelings, and behaviors that we see as erroneously attributed to biomechanical malfunctioning.

Further, and importantly, at no point do we intend to question the validity of the psychiatric diagnoses reported by interviewed women or those other people receive. We are not psychologists or psychiatrists, nor are we trained in psychology at the postgraduate level. We also agree and acknowledge that, when done correctly, psychological diagnoses are made based both on clinical training and evidence and can provide valuable assistance. Nor is it our intention to "lay diagnose" those interviewed for this book. Instead, we provide a space within which women who are otherwise unheard can share their own thoughts, beliefs, and experiences of trauma and the treatment they subsequently received. In some cases, women chose not to seek treatment, and their reasons also inform this book.

We have two reasons for suggesting that trauma, particularly as tied to structural violence, remains a stronger explanation than any of the various biomedical causes alone posited for the emotional and behavioral problems experienced by homeless citizens. The first is the failure of biopsych researchers to conclusively demonstrate their case with respect to any one of a number of other hypotheses that have been put forward. One need only look to the work of geneticists to illustrate this point.

That schizophrenia is a genetically based disorder has become something of a received dogma. This belief is predicated on the results of family and twin studies that purport to show the heritability of the condition (Cardno et al. 1999; Tsuang 2000). The failure of biopsych to produce a single gene or set of genes generally recognized as a cause or contributing factor to the development of schizophrenia has deterred neither biopsych researchers nor those similarly engaged in explaining other conditions from continuing their pursuits (Hughes and Peak 2013). In relation to the latter, the search for biopsych causes of the bipolar disorders (BPDs) is particularly instructive. Despite the existence of studies that purport to show "the high heritability" of BPD, researchers have had to admit that "few susceptibility genes have been identified and linkage and/or association studies have produced conflicting results" (Etain et al. 2008, p. 867). They have also had to acknowledge the role that social and environmental factors play in the development of BPD, particularly the experience of childhood trauma (Etain et al. 2008). The same results exist in relation to genetic research on anxiety disorders, which have also failed to yield fruitful results. Although biopsych proponents are firmly of the view that twin and association studies have adequately demonstrated the heritability of a predisposition to developing PTSD, generalized anxiety disorder, phobias, and so on, they have been forced to acknowledge their studies have been confounded by a number of methodological factors, including the inescapable fact of the contribution of environmental factors to the onset of these conditions (Norrholm and

Ressler 2009). The best they can suggest is that, in the case of PTSD, "its development *appears to be* mediated by both genetic and environmental contributions" (Norrholm and Ressler 2009, p. 272; emphasis added).[7] We are not alone in noting the lack of progress in this area and its import. In reviewing biopsychiatry's progress to date at least on the genetic front, Kenneth Kendler concludes,

> Despite our wishing so, individual gene variants of large effect appear to have a small to non-existent role in the etiology of major psychiatric disorders. We have clarified the role of genetic factors in comorbidity, elucidated development pathways and documented the importance of gene-environment correlation and interaction but our valued candidate genes produced quite limited insights into the nature of genetic risk for illness. While important in a number of ways, our heritability estimates provide no insight into underlying biological process and no guarantee that the syndrome is biologically coherent. (2013, p. 1066)

Reflecting on what future efforts might reveal, Kendler suggests that "the most pessimistic prediction that we will observe only a mess is unlikely," yet "discovering a highly coherent single pathway to illness also seems improbable. We can hope that the heterogeneity is not too great and the real level of illness not too hidden in the upper reaches of the mind-brain system" (Kendler 2013, p. 1066).

Finding support for the chemical imbalance hypothesis proves to be even more problematic than the search for candidate genes. Although frequently accepted by the public, evidence for the imbalance hypothesis has largely been drawn from random clinical trials that purport to show that a given drug produces better clinical outcomes than a placebo (Kirsch 2010). Extrapolating from such results, proponents argue that "response equals causation," a logic confounded by the fact that other clinical trials demonstrate the same drugs can have very little if any effect (France, Lysaker, and Robinson 2007). Further, other forms of treatment, in particular psychotherapy, can produce positive responses. Thus, as Christopher France and his colleagues suggest, if the same logic that underpins the imbalance hypothesis is employed, one might conclude that "a deficiency of psychotherapy causes depression" (2007, p. 412). In examining the commonly accepted claim that mental illness is a disease like any other, the psychologists George Albee and Justin Joffee note,

> One can search the literature without success for studies that have produced convincing evidence of a reliable objective organic cause of a "mental disease" (other than the old familiar ones like general paresis and senile dementia). For a hundred years it has been assumed that researchers are close to finding the biological cause of schizophrenia. But an overwhelm-

> ing amount of evidence suggests that the great majority of mental disorders are not a result of defective biology . . . [but] the brain processes involved in responding to stress and in learning atypical behaviors, thoughts, and emotions are normal, and there is no evidence that physical pathology is involved. (2004, p. 425)

We do not wish to suggest that biology does not play a role in mental disorders, nor is that what we intend to argue in this book. To the extent humans are all creatures of biology, biology must therefore play some role. Instead, we are arguing that the exact mechanisms by which mental disorders arise remain largely unknown, and trauma plays a much more significant role in the onset of mental disorders within certain populations than is generally credited.

The second reason we contend that trauma and other significant stressors are more viable answers to the question of what causes a degree of the mental and emotional distress labeled as psychiatric conditions is that trauma-related research consistently shows statistically significant correlations. For example, in a review of thirty-three studies, Maria Mauritz and colleagues (2013) found that prevalence rates of trauma and PTSD were significantly higher for those diagnosed with a serious mental illness. When the populations were weighted, the mean prevalence rates of interpersonal trauma for those with a serious mental health condition were 47 percent for physical abuse (with a range of 25 to 72 percent) and 37 percent for sexual abuse (range of 24 to 49 percent) (Mauritz et al. 2013). Some 30 percent were also diagnosed with PSTD (a range of 20 to 47 percent) (Mauritz et al. 2013).

The effects of trauma are particularly notable in relation to those mental health conditions most easily cast as the results of chemical imbalances, principally the category known as mood disorders. Of these, BPD is often seen as a fairly serious mental health condition because of the effects of its symptoms and its high rates of comorbidity with other diagnoses (Parker 2010). And yet, when looking at the volume of recent research on this form of supposed chemical imbalance, we find (1) studies have repeatedly shown high rates of interpersonal trauma in the histories of those diagnosed (Mowlds et al. 2010), (2) trauma is found to be a significant factor in the lives of those who develop comorbid conditions such as anxiety and substance abuse disorders, and (3) evidence has shown that chronic stressors over the life course can play an important role in the development of the depressive symptoms of BPD (Gershon, Johnson, and Miller 2013). Indeed, the connection between trauma and BPD is such that one group of biopsych researchers have concluded that "growing evidence suggests that incidences of childhood trauma are frequent and severe in bipolar disorder, probably affect the clinical expression of the disease in terms of suicidal behaviour and age at onset, and also have an insidious influence on the affective functioning of patients between episodes" (Etain et al. 2008, p. 867). Again, this conclusion supports the idea that more than biology is behind the development, for lack of a better word, of mental disorders.

Schizophrenia, another condition frequently attributed to a supposed chemical imbalance in levels of dopamine (a neurotransmitter) has been alternatively described as a "chronic terror syndrome" (Karon 2007, p. 127). In support of this contention, Bertram Karon points to the experience of combatants in World War II, who experienced schizophrenic symptoms as a product of the battlefield (Karon 2007). More recently, a wealth of data has come from noncombat situations that consistently demonstrate the relationship between forms of traumatic experience and both schizophrenia and schizoaffective disorders. For instance, significant correlations have been found between psychological trauma, particularly childhood sexual abuse, and psychotic symptoms (Freeman and Fowler 2009; Moskowitz et al. 2009). Perhaps not surprisingly, those with a history of trauma are more likely to develop paranoid hallucinations and feelings of being persecuted (Freeman and Fowler 2009). Research on schizoaffective disorder similarly reveals significant associations between childhood sexual abuse and auditory hallucinations (Hammersley et al. 2003). Changes in the brains of schizophrenic patients, often assumed to be of genetic or neurodevelopmental origin, have been shown to be linked to traumatic childhood experiences and subsequent chronic stressors (Read et al. 2001). And, perhaps most tellingly, in studies of schizophrenia, high rates of comorbidity have been shown to be linked to traumatic experience. In one such study, two-thirds of those diagnosed with a schizophrenia spectrum disorder reported "clinically significant trauma symptoms" (Lysaker and LaRocco 2008, p. 330). Individuals with experiences of trauma experienced greater levels of depression, anxious arousal, and hallucinations, leaving researchers to conclude that "trauma symptoms may be commonly experienced in schizophrenia and linked with the phenomenology of the disorder" (Lysaker and LaRocco 2008, p. 330), again lending support for the role of trauma in the development of clinical disorders.

The raft of studies and statistics cited is, of course, one form of support for our argument; however, the experiences of women like Joelle, Michelle, and a host of others whose stories inform the pages of this book are another form of empirical support. These are women who have been physically and sexually abused as children; been physically and sexually assaulted as adults; experienced fires, major illnesses, and tragic deaths; and inhabit highly adverse and sometimes physically dangerous spaces. Through the process of the clinical exam, they have also experienced the added indignity of having the signs of that suffering turned into forms of individual psychopathology. The understandable mental and emotional distress they bear is no longer about what was done to them but has become instead what is wrong inside of them.

Notes

1. An example would be cognitive behavioral therapy and dialectical behavioral therapy.

2. An example would be the practice of removing a woman's uterus to cure the condition then known as hysteria.

3. A stimulant and appetite suppressant, amphetamine is used to treat ADHD and narcolepsy (among other conditions). It functions by acting like adrenaline and stimulating the central nervous system, thus having an impact on the chemicals in the body. (See Centre for Addiction and Mental health at www.camh.ca/en/hospital/health_information for additional information on different psychopharmaceuticals and their use and effects.)

4. *Reaganomics* refers to the economic policies, based on supply-side theory, put forth by the former president of the United States Ronald Reagan. Proponents of supply-side theory argue that governments in lowering taxes on corporations will stimulate investment by and within industry, which will encourage production and, thus, control inflation and prices (Canto, Jones, and Laffer 1983).

5. For an example of a notable exception, see Lovell (1992).

6 Although he conflates psychiatry and psychology, Rose (1998) provides an illuminating discussion on the willingness of the psy sciences to lend their knowledge to other institutions.

7. Given that a diagnosis of PTSD is dependent on an individual having a prior traumatic experience (hence the term *posttraumatic stress*), the conclusion that environmental contributions may play a role is hardly earthshaking.

3

Trauma and Mental Illness

Lisa is a fifty-one-year-old woman residing in a homeless shelter in Pasadena, California. Although the shelter is variously described by other residents as "dirty," "crime ridden," and a "place where people go to die," Lisa, who has liver cancer and a host of other physical ailments, is grateful for the bed because it beats the alternative, of which she has had several years of experience. Since her husband died, Lisa has been sleeping in parks and on the streets, where she has been raped multiple times and physically assaulted. She has also had to spend time dodging police for unpaid tickets issued for panhandling and other nuisance offenses in order to avoid being sent to jail.

In discussing her time on the streets, Lisa describes it as "surviving." Today, she is physically and emotionally exhausted and says that "I'm too sick and I'm too tired. I don't think I could go back to surviving again." When the subject turns to how the public often views Lisa and other homeless citizens, she employs this word again: "People think homeless people are bums. Nah, they do what they have to do to survive."

Although Lisa had experienced an incredible amount of trauma in her life (more of which is discussed in later chapters), the unfortunate reality is that among homeless women, her stories, considered separately, were not unusual. Thousands and thousands of women share her stories. Some perhaps have not experienced violence and loss to the same extent as Lisa, but most had been sexually assaulted, beaten by strangers and intimates, watched loved ones die, been molested as children, and experienced parental abandonment and episodes of living in the streets (D'Ercole and Struening 1990; Jasinski et al. 2010; Wenzel, Koegel, and Gelberg 2000). In fact, one might reasonably suggest that few women living on the streets or in shelters do not have a history of trauma, and few can say they have not suffered violence, catastrophes, and significant loss beyond the mental, emotional, and physical difficulties that come with becoming and being homeless (Finfgeld-Connett 2010).

Some have suggested that the word *trauma* has become a "metaphor for almost anything unpleasant" (Hacking 1995, p. 183); however, in this book, we do not employ *trauma* in this colloquial sense. In the pages that follow, we use the term to refer to an experience that creates overwhelming feelings of fear, terror, helplessness, or horror. In the aftermath of such an event, individuals' sense of personal safety and security is damaged, often leaving them feeling anxious and depressed (Herman 1992). Those who have both the personal and social resources upon which to draw, including coping skills and supportive social networks, may in time experience resiliency and posttraumatic growth (Tedeschi and Calhoun 1995, 1996). However, many others who lack such supports remain in states of mild to severe depression, develop anxiety disorders or substance abuse issues, or experience a worsening of preexisting mental health issues (Joseph 2011; for an example, see Tyler, Melander, and Almazan 2010). They may also find themselves in interpersonal conflicts or with damaged relationships, experience difficulties with maintaining employment, develop suicidal ideation, or adopt self-harming behaviors, among other possible negative outcomes (Joseph 2011; Tyler, Melander, and Almazan 2010). In this chapter, we reveal the types of traumatic events women in the study have experienced, before considering the personal impact of these events on their present functioning. The chapter is organized in a seemingly chronological fashion: First, we present the traumatic experiences in childhood and adolescence, followed by those experienced in adulthood, as voiced by interviewees. Next, we present their resiliency and draw attention to their current situation, as described by the phrase "the trouble with normal." In this context, we provide some insight into the lives of these women and their personal histories to shed light on the harsh realities that have shaped their current situations. In doing so, we seek to show how the effects of trauma worsen in part by an individuals' belief that as a result of their experiences or their perceived inability to cope, they are not normal but instead damaged, thus creating a vicious circle within which many women remain trapped.

Terrible Things in Childhood and Adolescence

Researchers often discover that women living in shelters or in transitional housing frequently have histories of child abuse, abandonment, neglect, and other forms of maltreatment (Huey, Fthenos, and Hyrniewicz 2012, 2013;

Simons and Whitbeck 1991; Stein, Leslie, and Nyamathi 2002). Unfortunately, the women we interviewed in Los Angeles had suffered similar trauma, many of whom related stories of childhood neglect and maltreatment.

Of the various forms of suffering women experienced in childhood, one of the most common was parental abandonment. For example, Lidia's father had walked out on the family, leaving behind several children and a wife struggling with severe mental health issues. Lacking a second parent, Lidia and her siblings were placed in foster care after authorities discovered that then-thirteen-year-old Lidia had assumed the responsibility of looking after the younger children. "I had to be mommy," she says, "because mommy kept getting sick," and there were "no daddies in our life." Veronica has a similar story: "Let's see, I lost my father at seven. My mom went . . . in and out of hospitals, and I was left alone at the house . . . [and] she was very depressed and didn't know what to do or how to handle it." Like Lidia, Veronica was taking care of herself and her siblings until a neighbor "called social services and I was put in the foster care system." In other cases, mothers abandoned their children. Kenya's mother called her own mother (Kenya's maternal grandmother) to inform the older lady that she was walking out before leaving her infant daughter in a milk crate in a hotel room. Kenya's explanation for her mother's actions? "It was all because she wanted to get high and stay in the streets. Run with my father, shooting dope and all that kind of stuff." As evinced in Kenya's story, some women interviewed were born to alcoholic or addict parents who could not properly care for their children. Mina had a history of drug use that began at the age of eight when she was introduced to crack cocaine by her father, a drug dealer. When she was old enough, he put her to work selling crack. Other women began to use because drugs were part of their environment growing up, as Sammi explains: "I have a history of drugs since the age of eleven. My parents were both addicts. My dad was in and out of prison." Kerrie's father was a drug dealer and her mother a drug addict. She herself was "born on every type of drug" and abandoned by her parents after birth. She refers to her early life as "being left in the hospital."

Physical abuse is also a common element across many of the life stories we heard. Serena, now twenty-six, explains, in reference to her early life, "I grew up being abused every day, being hit, being dragged by my hair, being hit, being punched, being slammed." Teri says of the abuse she received at the hands of her father, "If I went to school like that today, they would put him in jail. I mean, I was beaten with a belt. I had welts and open wounds." Experiences of childhood physical abuse are often coupled with memories of witnessing other forms of domestic violence in the home. Sally confirms that her "first memory is seeing my dad beat the hell out of my mom." Similarly, Jane was forced to witness her mother's beatings at the hands of her stepfather. She describes these experiences as "her husband abused her and we were subjected to seeing it."

Many of the women interviewed had also been sexually abused as children. Most frequently, they would report experiences of being molested by family members—fathers, uncles, stepfathers, brothers, cousins—as well as by family friends. Cindy, for example, explained that at "like seven or eight years old and I was molested by my stepfather." When asked if she had ever experienced sexual abuse, Sarah replies, "My mother's brother molested me when I was a kid. I was maybe five or four." Joelle estimates that her experiences of sexual abuse began around the age of three with an uncle who "made me and my two little cousins, which were his sons, perform oral." She was also sexually abused by several other people, including a family friend. "Whenever [the adults would] get high on beer, weed . . . he would mess with me. All the time. Full blown sex. Shit, I was like in the first grade."

As a result of abuse, neglect, abandonment, and other forms of maltreatment, some of the women were placed in foster care. Kim is one: "I was taken away from my parents when I was nine years old and was in foster care until I turned eighteen." Another woman, Charlene, entered foster care in California as an adolescent. Once in the system, she was abused by men in three different foster homes. Twenty-year-old Abby had been in six different foster homes after being "born into the system." She says she was moved around because "a lot of the homes I went into, the people were abusive." Teresa is understandably bitter over her years of abuse within foster care. Between herself and her siblings, she says, "We were in foster homes for years. I also got molested there . . . [because] they all do it." Teresa, in making her rather sweeping statement—"they all do it"—acknowledges the systemic violence structuring the foster care system, despite best intentions in its purpose and design. The realities underlying the conditions due to which children are placed in foster care and then their experiences in foster care represent structural violence. Experiences that define childhood then resonate with and shape the lives of the women living on Skid Row. Other women were placed in relatives' homes. These placements were often unstable, with children being moved among relatives' homes. Tina, who was one of those who had been bounced among relatives, describes her first "stable home" as the shelter in which she presently resides.

As adolescents, many youth living within troubled parental or foster homes ended up on the streets: some by running away, others being kicked out of their homes, and several joining street gangs, often in search of love and support. Joelle's first stint of homelessness began as an adolescent when her mother kicked her out of the house for being gay. Kathy ended up on the streets when she was kicked out of the family home for being pregnant at fourteen. Living on the streets of Los Angeles at fourteen, she was, in her own words, "like a street urchin." "Have you ever seen children of the night where they go around and try to scoop up the kids on the street at night?" Kathy asks. "Like that. But I never got scooped up." Serafina was scooped up, but by street gangs with whom she associated until she watched another girl "[get] her brains blown out right in front of me."

Although much of the childhood trauma reported centered on abuse and neglect, other forms of traumatic experience were also revealed. Principal among these was the death of a parent or other significant person. Loni was raised by her grandparents after they realized her own parents, who were both drug addicts, could not care for her. Although she never knew her mother, she maintained relations with her father and would sometimes visit his family home. These visits ended when she was fifteen and he was found dead after a heroin overdose in a bus station. Of her father's death, she says, "They told too much." Loni then illustrates what "too much" entailed:

> They showed me the bus station. They told me about the guy that knew he was dying, how he heard him take his last breath. Then they told me about the letter he had in his wallet for me. It said, "I hope to be able . . . I don't want to do this anymore. I want to be there for you. I want to be part of your family and I love you very much." He did too much and he died.

Loni's story, like many others, reveals the pain embedded in the trauma and the associated irrecoverable loss.

Speaking with Freda reveals yet another pathway to mental and emotional issues that can continue to haunt women throughout their lives. Like Joelle, Vanessa, and a handful of other lesbian women who participated in this study, Freda was victim of homophobia from an early age, originating from both her family and community, in another manifestation of structural violence. These experiences had a devastating impact on her identity and self-esteem. In Freda's case, she was raised within a Southern Baptist family whose beliefs about homosexuality reinforced her sense of otherness. As a result, she learned to suppress her feelings and her identity. Reflecting on this time, Freda adds, "I knew I was gay. I knew I was gay at seven, and I'm going to church every Sunday hearing [that] I'm going to burn in hell."

Terrible Things in Adulthood

Relative to women in the general population, women without permanent housing frequently experience significantly higher rates of trauma during their adult lives. From domestic violence to sexual assault, incarceration, and the loss of custody of their children, the stories of homeless women all too often reflect deeply painful experiences (Barrow and Laborde 2008; Browne and Bassuk 1997; Huey, Fthenos, and Hryniewicz 2012; Jasinski et al. 2010).

In Los Angeles, a majority of the women interviewed had been physically and sexually abused by intimate partners. Karen, discussing her former partner, explains: "The first time he did it, I forgave him because I was in love with him and I thought it would never happen again. The second time it happened, he beat me so bad, I was in the hospital for a month and half." Her ex is now serving a life sentence: "He's doing life now because, as it turns out, I wasn't the only one." Tina's partner "would beat the shit of me almost to where I could barely move." Susan spoke of escaping a husband who would "beat me and my kids." She explains that "he'd be gone for a week, two weeks, and then when he came home, he'd wake the kids up, and they'd have to sit up and watch him beat me up." Johnna's former partner was also her pimp: "He was horrible to me. Black eyes, busted lips. Beat up. Traveling from place to place. Paying all the bills just solely through prostitution." Melanie got married at seventeen and says of that time, "I was abused for eight years by my husband . . . two broken jaws. A lot of black eyes. I had stitches in my lips. Cut off fingers." When asked about domestic violence, Aisha relates that her "second baby daddy hit me in the ear with a brick."

Some women reported having been physically assaulted by nonintimate partners. In some instances, the individual was previously known to them, as was the case with Eva, who was assaulted on the street by a man she knew: "I was just walking to my destination, and the guy punched me in the face because I didn't want to have sex with him." She explains: "We was in a room one time and I left. I pulled a prank and I made him pay for the room and everything. He was pissed off when I took off." Sherry was "rolled" by street friends who knew she had money and was too weak to defend herself:

> I was coming down off of heroin. I was going through a really bad withdrawal. I was weak and . . . basically the people that know you, who know where you going to pick up your drugs, and they see you coming and they know you have money on you. And I wasn't able to . . . I wasn't able to defend myself and they took my money, um, pretty much bashed my face in and broke my jaw.

Other women had also been assaulted during the commission of a robbery, but by complete strangers. One such story was Ella's. Fifty-eight, and with years of life spent on the streets, Ella had recently been robbed, and the evidence was apparent in what appeared to be a seriously damaged eye: "I was going to the cigarette house when they approached me." With only a quarter on her to buy a cigarette, she was attacked by a group of people, one of whom "kicked me in my eye with steel-toed boots."

The experience of sexual assault among the women of Los Angeles is depressingly common. Fifty-eight-year-old Ella had been both physically and sexually victimized. One assault occurred while she was performing sex work in the Skid Row District. Ella explains, "I got into a car with a guy. We were 'dating.' He grabbed me around my neck and just choked me until I went out." She doesn't remember much of what happened until "I woke up in a puddle of my own boo boo and urine." Shana had also been raped while working the streets:

> Short version: I got into a van one night with a guy and he seemed like a really nice guy and he drove us to an alley. And now the person I got in the car with was now Mr. Hyde, no more Mr. Jekyll. I reached out to grab the door and he pulled the locks off. He pulled out a knife and tried to force me to perform oral sex on him.

Sandra had a similar experience while walking down a street. She was grabbed at knifepoint by an unknown man and forced into his van, where she was sexually assaulted. Aisha was also attacked by a stranger, who pulled her into bushes with a gun to her head. Recalling the experience, she speaks of being in fear for her life: "He told me he was going to shoot me." Although most cases of sexual assault involved one perpetrator, several of the women reported having been raped by multiple perpetrators. When asked about her experiences of violence, Lori replies, "I got raped at sixteen by five guys."

The experience of witnessing significant violence as an adult was another common theme in interviews. Devon, who was newly homeless, said that shortly after arriving in the Skid Row area, "I saw this man get killed here. . . . They were fighting." When one man was punched, she adds, "he hit his head on the concrete." What especially shocked Devon was the rapaciousness of the onlookers: "Before he could hit the ground, they's checking his pockets."

As with the example provided by Serafina's story, some of the violence witnessed and experienced by the women in this study was gang related. Mercedes was similarly involved in gang activities as a young woman, activities which nearly cost her to lose her eyesight when a truck she was in was shot at by a rival gang member:

> They shot behind the bit of the truck I was in with my boyfriend. The bullet went in between our heads and we were sitting close together. It hit the

> windshield, and then when I was looking like that, it went between our heads and the glass went into our eyes. That was really traumatic for me because a doctor told me if I was to move my eyes to the left or right I would cut up my eyes. He didn't even know if I would be able to see again. . . . I went to UCLA [University of California, Los Angeles] the next day, [and] they picked the glass out of my eyes.

Trish was nearly killed in a drive-by shooting five months earlier when she and her boyfriend were talking to the target of a gang-related feud: "Me, him, and this other guy in the apartments were talking, and his wife was there . . . [and] he was related in gangs . . . and out of nowhere some guy comes and starts shooting. I don't know how, but I wasn't shot. The bullets were coming towards me. They were all around where I was sitting." The acquaintance, whom she described as a "nice man" who would bring stuffed toys for her daughter, was killed. "In the morning, walking out . . . his body was still there."

Not all traumatic experiences reported directly entailed physical or sexual violence. Almost a third of the women interviewed had experienced the loss of custody of their children, and most spoke of how agonizing this process was for them. One of the most heart-wrenching stories came from Michelle, a thirty-one-year-old African American woman residing in a shelter in Skid Row. Running out of resources and unable to find a family shelter to take her and her two boys, aged six and two, she made a difficult decision. She placed the oldest one with his father and surrendered her youngest child into foster care. "I actually took him in myself. . . . I told them it was an emergency and I wouldn't be able to take care of him. I wanted to give them reassurance that I wanted to get both of them back." Wiping away her tears, she says, "I have to do this until I can get it situated."

Women not uncommonly reported having experienced the death of someone they were close to, such as an intimate partner or a child. Aisha's husband had only recently passed away from liver cancer. For Aisha, as well as for a handful of other women, the death of their loved one was also the catalyst for their homelessness. When Amanda's husband died, she was left financially destitute. Only a month after his death, she found herself moving into a homeless shelter. Talking to the interviewer, she tries to be emotionally strong but acknowledges, "It's pretty difficult for me right now. I haven't gotten over this grief yet. I just focus on how to get my life back together without him. It's kinda hard [crying]."

Many of the women had also been incarcerated. Their carceral experiences ranged from spending a few hours in police lockup for unpaid tickets to years in state or federal correctional facilities for serious offenses. Each found the experience highly unpleasant, and some left custody feeling traumatized. Gina was among the latter. She had joined a gang, the Crips, in the San Fernando Valley and began dealing drugs. She says she learned the hard way that "bad stuff happens to you when you're gangbanging," including "getting killed or jail." In Gina's case, she ended up serving two years in a state correctional facility. What was already a bad situation grew worse following a fight with a correctional officer, whereupon she was placed in solitary confinement for a year. "You go absolutely berserk," she relates. "I used to count bricks. There was rats. I would have to block the door, so the rats wouldn't come in and chew up everything." Reflecting on this for a moment, Gina quickly adds, "I'm not going back." Joelle held her last regular job in 1990. From 1990 to 2013 she made her living through drug dealing. As a result, she explains, her "life has been kind of a mess," with stints of going "back and forth to jail." She has also served two prison sentences for violence-related offenses. Her violence stems from anger, she says. "Going to jail, a lot of my anger comes too from that. Going to jail a lot of times for things that . . . I won't say that I didn't do it, but it wasn't serious enough to give me the type of time that I did, and to be around the type of people I had to be around." What makes Joelle particularly angry is that "sometimes it seemed like nobody cared."

Less frequently, women spoke of dealing with the stresses of major illness or of being involved in a devastating fire. In relation to health problems, Lynn has been positive for the human immunodeficiency virus (HIV) for thirty-three years, which she says is "a long fucking time to live with the virus. I'm fifty-five now, and I've had a heart attack and lived with that shit." She adds, "I don't know how much time I have. So I have to do the best I can do to get the most out of my life. And this isn't it. Living at the shelter isn't it." Carole was infected with human papilloma virus (HPV) while working in the adult film industry at a time when actors weren't routinely tested for HPV. As a result, "I ended up with cervical cancer and I had to have almost all of my cervix removed." A few women had been victims of motor vehicle accidents that left them with serious injuries. One was Aisha, who is on disability after being hit by a car: "I got four pins, those titanium pins, on each side in my pelvis, and I got one on my ass bone holding me together." Lilly had been caught in a hotel fire. She had realized that a portion of the building was on fire and, on instinct, ran down the halls banging on doors, yelling at people to leave. In her efforts to save lives, Lilly received severe burns on her hands and arms. When Kay's house caught on fire, three of her children were killed. This accident precipitated a seventeen-year downward spiral into alcoholism and addiction, during which Kay spent the better part of those years literally living on or near St. Julian Street in Skid Row.

A Miserable State

Regardless whether a woman had experienced a traumatic or otherwise significantly stressful event at an earlier point in her life—that is, forms of direct or indirect (structural) violence—each participant had experienced the pains of becoming and being homeless. The pathways into homelessness were as diverse as the women interviewed. About a third were newly homeless as a result of the 2008 financial crisis and the continuing stagnant job market in the United States. This group included teachers, low-level managers, bookkeepers, and nursing students and college students. Susan was fired from her job at a law firm for needing time off to deal with child-care issues. Becca could not graduate with her nursing credentials because she could not pay off student loans from her private college. Sixty-nine-year-old Susan lost both her job and her home when she was let go as the caretaker for an elderly man. For others, family disputes, including domestic violence, precipitated their flight into homelessness. Juliet, sixty-one and homeless for four months, could not find family members to take her in because "I have a clutter problem." Asked to elaborate, she explains that she had spent all of the money received from a legal settlement on items that filled her house, causing family members to say, "You're a hoarder," and to deny her accommodation when her situation became financially precarious. Donna's homelessness came as a result of her addiction to alcohol and drugs, which led to disputes with roommates over her partying: "I started having too many people in, because you get lonely there. So you have friends come in and out, smoking weed, drinking." Some women, such as thirty-one-year-old Lana, attributed their homelessness to ongoing mental health problems. Lana says, "I tried to work, [but] it didn't work out. I had a bunch of nervous breakdowns. I couldn't handle [the] pressure because of all the posttraumatic stuff when I was younger." Lee, who was repeatedly sexually abused as a child, identifies depression, a condition she had hid from friends and family for decades, as the cause of her homelessness. Once homeless, Lee's depression worsened to the point where she became suicidal:

> You know, when it all went . . . I had never been in that position. I don't know people in that position. Then all of a sudden, I get off the bus in Long Beach, and I'm looking around thinking, "Where do you want to go?" and I have nowhere to go. I slept for the first time in my life in some apartment complex laundry room and it's a horrible thing. It was a bad thing. It was the worst thing I'd ever experienced in my life. I don't know where to go. Where do I sleep? [Starts crying.] . . . I have nowhere to go and I'm scared out here. I know that suicide isn't of God, but it's like I'm not doing this because I want to, but because you don't have any place for me to sleep.

Lee's words here demonstrate just how dire and hopeless her situation felt.

Prior to coming to a shelter, several of the women had spent time sleeping in cars or sleeping "rough."[1] Donna, for example, when first evicted from her final apartment, had started sleeping in her car until it was eventually impounded for unpaid tickets. "You got no place, you got no car, puts you in the streets. So then you're living in drug houses." Ella had been sleeping under the freeway with some of her street friends. Others had slept in the city's streets and alleys, sometimes in tents or on mattresses, often with only a few blankets. Karen had been relatively fortunate in that she had been able, to pitch her tent in an acquaintance's backyard, where she would be less exposed, as was the case with Sandy, who had set her tent up on a city sidewalk, or Lisa, who had been tenting in a park. Before coming to a shelter, Teneka too had been sleeping on a mattress in an alley. When asked if it had been dangerous for her to be a woman alone and exposed in such a vulnerable space, she replied, "Oh yeah, it was very, very dangerous. There was shootings and everything." Sixty-eight-year-old Dottie addressed the issue of female vulnerability directly while discussing the two and a half weeks she spent sleeping "on that cement over there [pointing to a space behind the shelter]." As an eighteen-year veteran of the Skid Row area, she was keenly aware of the fact that "a lot of women down here, they're sleeping on the streets, [and] they get raped," so she took "the little blankets that I had" and found a space to sleep where "there's security guards, so this way nobody's bothering you." Indeed, she found her own form of pseudo-protection despite being exposed and unsafe on the streets.

Living in a shelter can be, and often is, an undeniably stressful time. Privacy and personal space are unattainable, and there is no autonomy. Several of the women complained about having to follow rules they felt were largely arbitrary. Forty-three-year-old Patty said, "It's like being in jail, but we do what we have to do so that we have a roof over our head." Patty's comparison of living in a shelter to living in prison suggests that the "freedom" tied to being on the streets, in comparison to incarceration, may be the only advantage of not being incarcerated these women experience.

Although some women are fortunate enough to stay at the Women's Center or other facilities in Los Angeles that provide individual rooms, most were placed in either dorm-style accommodations with dozens of other women or in shared rooms. At Carole's shelter, she lives in a room with six other women. Laura went inside Carole's room and it resembled a squat, with mattresses on the floor for six women and stuff strewn about because of a lack of storage. One resident had tried to cheer up her section of the room by taping up pictures from yoga magazines and a few leaves she had found. Not surprisingly, Carole paints a depressing picture of her shelter.

She sees herself as living "in a tight space with people that don't care anymore . . . [and] it brings your spirits down. There are people that are here just waiting to die. They do. It's sad. It makes everyone else sad." She adds, "And it makes other people think, 'Maybe I'm here too just waiting to die.'"

Almost a year later, the team returned to this shelter and heard depressingly similar stories from some of the new women we met. Quadra, a recovering alcoholic, had recently relapsed when exposed to the alcohol and drug use of other residents, as well as to tensions and conflicts among roommates. One such recent conflict had escalated into minor violence. Quadra explains, "This place is hell on wheels. I have to fight to stay alive in here. Safe. And mentally well." Zoe is petrified of this same facility. She describes it as "very stressful [because] they put you in with a person that's crazy, and they could do something to you while you're sleeping. They just let everybody run around like crazy, and I'm sleeping with a stranger, and I have to watch myself because I don't know if they're going to kill me while I'm asleep." As a result of her fears, she has developed a weird rash that she blames on "anxiety." Of her stay at this facility, she concludes, "It's nerve wracking . . . it's like being in a prison." Even more discouraging was the presence of several women that we had met here, at the shelter, nearly nine months earlier. These women had been convinced at the time that they were well on the way to moving into permanent housing. Only one of those women, Elise, had done so, but when she became sick with liver cancer, she lost her housing. Now back at the shelter, she feared what would happen to her if she lost her meager accommodations at this place—described by others as "hellish"—and ended up on the streets again. In her lilting Tennessee accent, she ponders this possibility: "Anything I can do to stop it, I'm gonna do. I don't want to die in the park. You know what I'm sayin'?"

Further some of the shelters in Los Angeles have hygiene problems, including scabies and bedbugs. Women related stories of washrooms where menstrual blood, urine, or feces had been liberally splashed on toilets, floors, and walls. Donna, who is living in the same shelter as Carole, says that despite the fact that case managers were supposed to verify the cleanliness of the rooms, bedbugs were still prevalent. "Every room I go into, I have to clean the walls. They have boogers on there. They had everything on there." To deal with such poor living conditions, Kesha has hidden a bottle of bleach, which she uses on a daily basis to clean her bed and the surrounding walls.

Women residing in either women-only or mixed-gender shelters experienced specific and shared challenges. In the women-only shelters, several participants spoke of feeling they were in a combative environment with individuals who were prone to "drama." For example, Aisha states, "Up here on the floor, we got sixty, seventy women in here. . . . What do we got? . . .

Estrogen? . . . Too much of that going around. It's too much drama." Similarly, other women referred to "a lot of [verbal] attacks" and residents "complain[ing] about the least little thing" to each other. Lilly says that she has been using the shelter so long that she no longer has the drive to get out of her present situation: "A lot of it could be [that] this situation is making me depressed. I don't have that spirit I used to have. They're making me nuts. One hundred and sixty-one girls in one room? For as long as I've been here? It's a lot. A lot of drama, a lot of fighting . . . too much of everything." Her words reveal how living in the all-female shelter took all her energy, leaving her without the needed "spirit" to try to better her situation.

Problems were also cited in the mixed-gender shelters. Ramona, who had been kicked out of her family home when it was discovered she was pregnant, bounced around friends' houses and shelters. Of the mixed-gender shelters she has stayed in, she relates, "I was sexually harassed there all the time and I hated it." Carly had a violent encounter in one shelter, when she had reacted badly to a man touching her without her consent. Recently, she had been almost hit by a flying needle as she walked past a male in a hallway. She is now eager to move out of her Skid Row shelter to a place where "there's nobody throwing syringes at you as you walk by . . . as they pull it out of their arm." She then cracks a joke, before acknowledging that the experience has "fucked [her] up."

One of the most stressful aspects of residing in many shelters is their "limited stay" policies, which force women to leave after the maximum period of stay has been reached. Michelle is one of the women affected by such a policy: at the time of the interview, she is on her second stint at the same shelter she was previously forced to leave, and time is running out on her second stay. She is also keenly aware of the fact that despite her best efforts to land a job, her first shelter stay resulted in nothing more than her return to the streets with her two children in tow, and so she has little hope that the results of this second stay will be any different. Callie is another individual who is feeling this particular form of stress. In describing the burden these policies place on women, she reveals, "Sometimes being able to get into a shelter, it helps. But when you can't get in somewhere or you're forced to move into another direction, you have to be flexible and it's very draining."

Although we visited shelters and transitional housing facilities throughout the county of Los Angeles, much of our work was centered in the Skid Row District. For some of the women, particularly those who became newly homeless as a result of financial difficulties, entering Skid Row was itself a traumatic experience. Several describe themselves as being "shocked" by the poverty, addiction, and violence they saw for the first time. Indeed, one or two state they had never heard of Skid Row before they came and so were mentally and emotionally unprepared for what they would find. As in the vignette that opens this book, one of these women is Nikki. Another is Devon, who thought she was pretty streetwise until she arrived on Skid Row: "When I came, this is the first time in my life when I saw so many women with black eyes. There's a women's center down the street, and at one time there was six women in there with black eyes." Devon is shocked at the violence directed toward women in this community: "I've never seen that in my life. That's what they do here [shakes head]."

What Doesn't Kill You . . .

In one of the final essays he wrote before his death, the author Christopher Hitchens (2012) delivers what can only be called a fierce rebuke of one of the most famous bromides found in the English language: "What doesn't kill you makes you stronger." Grappling with the miseries of a terminal illness and the often brutal treatments taken to battle it, Hitchens notes that this expression was one he found himself "not saying with quite the same conviction as I once used to" (p. 59). His reluctance to put much stock in this phrase came from the fact that he now knew very well the physical toll that his battle with cancer was taking on his body. What Hitchens had discovered, and what many of us who study the effects of trauma know all too well, is that "there are all too many things that could kill you, don't kill you, and then leave you considerably weaker" (p. 60).

The effects of traumatic events on the individual are well documented. Researchers know, for instance, that early trauma in the lives of children can have a significant, long-term impact on their developing brains and those parts of the endocrine system that govern responses to external stressors (Heitt, Graham, and Nemeroff 1999). One such notable effect is how, if exposed to danger, the body can become sensitized to potential threats in the environment, retriggering the flight-or-fight sequence (Bloom 2009). The more this sequence activates, the more sensitized the individual can become, leading to a chronic state of hyperarousal manifested in crippling feelings of anxiety (Bloom 2009). Researchers have also demonstrated that exposure to trauma can affect individual cognition, particularly in how people view themselves, others, and their environment. For example, child abuse (Browne and Winkelman 2007), intimate partner violence (Jones, Hughes, and Unterstaller 2001), physical assault (Johansen et al. 2007), sexual assault (Ullman et al. 2007), and the witnessing of domestic violence by children (Herrenkohl et al. 2008) are each linked to emotional impairments and cognitive distortions associated with perceptions of self (self-blame, self-criticizing), sensitivity to potential threat, and feelings of helplessness and hopelessness.[2] Distorted perceptions and beliefs are further associated with feelings of depression and anxiety, suicidal ideation, eating disorders, and PTSD symptomology, among other symptoms of distress (Elzy et al. 2013; Heitt, Graham, and Nemeroff 1999).

In Los Angeles, some women spoke openly about the emotional impact of the various forms of trauma they had experienced. Annie is carrying survivor's guilt following a series of deaths she has experienced. Speaking of these losses, she says, "I can get emotional. Last year, about five of my street family died and one is still is a coma. We don't really know what happened and nobody even seems to care." Then, she adds, "There has been more deaths. My ex-husband died. And another boyfriend died before that. I've got a lot of guilt." Meanwhile, Kathy locates the root of her feelings of shame and low self-worth in her experiences of being sexually molested as a child. "I'm a textbook for the stuff that happened, the behaviors. Someone flipped my switch too early as far as sex and sexual feelings . . . [and] I carried a lot of shame for that." For years, Kathy never spoke about the sexual abuse or the "barrage of feelings" she carried with her: "I didn't tell anybody. . . . You can't talk about sexual molesting. I mean there's so much of it that affects you." Olivia recognizes how the trauma witnessed or experienced among women living on Skid Row can also have lasting effects: "Some of the people out here got real mental issues, but they didn't have 'em before they came here. I took a girl to lunch. The next time I seen her, she was talking to a tree." Of all the women who discussed the connections they had made between traumatic events and subsequent emotional distress, Maria puts the matter the most succinctly: "Everyone that I've talked to in this program has been sexually abused at one time in their life while they were children. Why do you think we're all so fucked up in the head? [Laughs.] Why do you think we're all shoving drugs down our throats? Every single one of them."

Throughout the course of a lifetime, a significant number of people will experience events that have the potential to leave them in varying states of mental and emotional distress. Over time, and by drawing on inner resources, positive coping strategies, and social supports, people can see these effects dissipate, a process termed *resilience* (Joseph 2011; Rutter 1987). As the famous Nietzschean bromide suggests, some of us may in fact even emerge from an ordeal not only feeling more positive and emotionally and mentally stronger but also having a new sense of purpose (Tedeschi and Calhoun 1995). However, the ability to experience resiliency or posttraumatic growth is not a given, and thus many are not simply able to "just get over" mental and emotional distress. This inability is particularly acute in the case of homeless women, many of whom come from environments in which they were not taught positive coping strategies, they were disadvantaged by structural violence, or there was a profound lack of individual and social support. Thus, when Michael Ungar writes of individual resiliency as a personal and cultural process largely "dependent upon the capacity and willingness of people's social ecologies to meet [their] needs" (2013, p. 256), one can see why many of the women in this study cannot develop positive coping mechanisms that are sufficient to help them overcome histories of significant mental, physical, and emotional neglect and abuse.

When individuals fail to overcome traumatic experiences and, worse still, develop negative coping strategies as a result, such as depending on drugs, alcohol, and unhealthy relationships, the result is a sharpening of the cognitive distortions engendered by the traumatic experience or even the development of new ones. This dynamic can be seen in the words of those women who admitted to feeling trapped in ongoing cycles of self-blame, depression, negative coping, and despair. Kathy, who has spent most of her life dimming the pain of sexual abuse and years spent on the streets, is now recovering from addictions to alcohol and methamphetamine (crystal meth). She was fortunate to have recently found a therapeutic program that she felt was really helping her. Of her struggle to overcome her past, she says, "I'm packing the most unhealthy skills ever in my tool bag." As a result, "I just didn't get it. And for a long time I felt so ashamed. I felt so bad about myself. I just couldn't understand what was wrong. I felt that we had this round world, and I was a square peg trying to fit in there." This idea, that she did not fit into the so-called normal world and there was something somehow abnormal about her, was a recurring theme in several interviews.

Although some, such as Kathy, feel able to undo the mental baggage of the past, others live with a sense of hopelessness. One individual clearly suffering from a form of despair over what she perceives as her inability to move beyond the past is Moorea, who lost custody of her four children. When asked what her future looks like, she replies,

> MOOREA: I hate to say this . . . I don't want to speak in negativity because if it comes to pass . . . but . . . it looks gloomy. I'm finished. It's all downhill.
>
> LAURA: Really? Why do you think that?
>
> MOOREA: The four Cs: choices, chances, conditions, and consequences. I made poor choices in my younger years, and I'm dealing with the consequences of those choices.

Similarly, Meredith, a fifty-six-year-old woman who has been homeless for five years, sees herself as living in a downward spiral due to her addictions to alcohol, cocaine, and marijuana. She describes herself as being "like a crab in a bucket": "Every time I try to get out, I get pushed back. The illness overpowers everything." For her, drugs make life more tolerable: "It makes you have the 'fuck its,' and the 'fuck its' is easier than reality." Whereas Meredith frames her substance abuse as an illness over which she had no choice, which makes her feel helpless over it, Natalie sees her alcoholism as something over which she had a choice and yet remained unaccountably helpless to understand or control: "I just chose not to be sober . . . [and] then I started doing other drugs . . . [and] I don't know why." Although Natalie acknowledges she has been dealing with recurring memories of sexual abuse by a favorite uncle, of her drinking she says, "I don't know what's wrong with me [crying]. I feel like I don't even know me anymore." She doubts her ability to remain sober and turn her life around because each day, when she searches for a reason to let go of the guilt and shame she is carrying, "I start drinking and I forget about the reason." Zaidie, who at twenty-two has survived abuse, foster care, and a life of gangbanging on the streets, feels unable to cope. She deals with her past by consciously repressing memories of it but acknowledges that "at the end of the day that pain, those thoughts, is still there."

The Trouble with Normal

When comparing themselves to what they perceived to be personal or societal standards of normalcy, the women interviewed repeatedly revealed they felt uniquely inferior for "failing to measure up" and thus carried with them burdens of shame and guilt for their perceived inability to function "normally." In discussing these feelings of inadequacy, as became apparent, most had never considered the possibility that they have actually been experiencing very normal symptoms of distress, common to any individual dealing with unresolved trauma or struggling within adverse conditions. What was surprising was that despite the fact that the majority had seen one or more mental health professionals over the course of their lives—indeed, many were receiving some form of mental health treatment at the time of their interview—only a small handful had ever been told in a clinical setting that they were behaving in very normal ways for someone who had experienced the type of trauma they had been through. In fact, several were themselves surprised to hear us point out that it was not at all unusual for, say, a victim of sexual assault, to develop feelings of anxiety, to become hypervigilant around strangers, or to feel uncomfortable in entering or leaving certain spaces.

To help both the researchers and women being interviewed draw clearer connections between their environment, their experiences, their unique personalities, and their present issues, including how unresolved trauma might manifest in troubling thoughts, emotions, and behaviors, team members began to employ the phrase "you're normal for where you're at." In doing so, we sought to redefine normal. One of the problems with the colloquial use of *normal* is that it refers to those things that are seen as typical in ordinary, routine, nonchaotic contexts. In such conditions, seven-year-olds are not sexually abused by their parents, women are not beaten on a daily basis, adolescents are not taught how to sell drugs or their bodies, nor are individuals randomly attacked for their gender, their sexuality, or the color of their skin. Thus, a use of the word *normal* that does not include a recognition of, and accounting for, the fact that the world, and our experiences of it, are highly contingent phenomenon, is one that is both useless as a meaningful construct and damaging to those who suffer from the fact they do not live in ordinary, routine, nonchaotic worlds.

And yet the whole edifice of the psy sciences is built on a rather static conception of normalcy and the illusory belief that meaningful statements can be made based not on contingency but on standardization to a so-called norm (Frances 2013). When women deviate from the expected norm, as individuals with significant unhealed trauma invariably do, the psy sciences tell them their suffering may be less than normal. Biopsychiatry, more specifically, says that the manifestations of this suffering are products of pathological processes within their purportedly diseased or malfunctioning minds. In essence, then, those individuals who already feel they are not normal, and suffer more as a result of their own perceived inadequacies and shame, have their worst fears confirmed by medical authorities, including those who hold the power to prescribe.

Notes

1. *Rough*, a term used in the homeless community and research literature, refers to sleeping outside or unsheltered.

2. Some studies suggest that these emotional and cognitive effects can be very similar for those who are experiencing the death of a loved one, and, as a result, they report a significant number of PTSD symptoms (Gold et al. 2005).

4

Encountering the Medical Profession

For decades, fifty-two-year-old Suzall has been struggling with the effects of trauma manifested as chronic depression and suicidal ideations. Like many survivors of childhood sexual abuse, Suzall reported her abuse to her parents and received no validation, support, or treatment. Instead, she was blamed for her own victimization because "nobody wants to hear it." So she learned to mask her feelings, becoming "just good at covering it up." "I was real good," she adds. "You'd think I was the happiest person in the world." Therefore, family and friends were purportedly surprised when they later found out that she had been on the 710 freeway getting ready to end her life.

In the end, Suzall, a religious woman, chose not to jump. Instead she walked out of her life by taking a bus to Long Beach, California, where she ended up sleeping in the laundry rooms of apartment buildings. Still struggling with suicidal feelings, she eventually sought help and was admitted to UCLA Harborview, where, for the first time in her life, at the age of fifty-one, she first received both a diagnosis for her condition—"mood disorder, depression, and suicidal," she says—and a treatment regimen. Suzall is fortunate in that she was diagnosed and first treated in a facility that, upon release, referred her to a comprehensive mental health center that marries drug treatment with psychotherapy and group classes. As a result, she is one of the minority of women in this study whose diagnosis was understood as being linked to significant trauma and treated as such.

Indeed, once upon a time, individuals entering a psychiatrist's office had a reasonable expectation of seeing something that currently would be more at home in a museum: an analyst's couch. Patients would be expected to recline, or at the very least to sit on the couch, and for fifty minutes or so begin the process of pouring out the contents of their psyches into the listening ear of a largely silent individual with a notepad. Within that environment, patients were encouraged to discuss not only traumatic events of the past but also family dysfunction, interpersonal relations, and anything else that might potentially have a bearing on shaping their mental and emotional lives. But now, not only have the accoutrements of the therapeutic exchange been altered—the couch replaced with office chairs, and the notepad swapped for a prescription pad—but the content of the session is also vastly different. Today, assuming that the diagnosis comes from a psychiatrist rather than a primary care physician, the individuals seeking help will likely spend far less than fifty minutes discussing their problems. Instead, most of that time will be taken up with answering questions about the nature of their symptoms and, if (when) a prescription is given, how their symptoms are responding to the drugs prescribed.

What is occurring through the exchanges held in the modern-day doctor's office is a clinical examination of the patient by an expert whose goal is, simply put, to reduce what are perceived to be unhealthy thoughts, feelings, and behaviors into a standardized diagnosis: a manifestation of the power of biopsychiatry to diagnose and thus to define an individual's problem and its origins, nature, and scope. This process does not necessarily include the taking of a detailed patient history. From a biopsych perspective, mental illness is considered predominantly biological in origin, and environmental and social factors have little bearing on what is seen as organic disease. The signs of trauma and other adversity—the residue of one's history—are thus redefined as markers of neurochemical malfunctioning.

In the pages that follow, we examine the avenues through which women came to receive a psychiatric diagnosis. Then, drawing on a handful of individual stories, we explore how signs of distress came to form the diagnoses that the women had received. From here, we turn the discussion to the issue of identity and how women have variously rejected or adopted, in whole or in part, the labels attached to a given diagnosis, and what benefits, if any, such labels may confer. In the final section, we discuss the issue of biopsychiatry's continuing misattribution of the causes of women's suffering.

Entering the System

Most homeless women use the healthcare services provided either directly through their shelters or through the network of nonprofit agencies that dot the landscapes of impoverished spaces.[1] For example, larger shelters frequently offer both medical (general practitioners and nurse practitioners) and mental health services (psychologists, social workers, and counselors) on-site. These services may also include access to a staff psychiatrist, although Laura observed that shelters are more likely to offer psychiatric treatment to clients through off-site arrangements with a psychiatric practice or multifunction mental health agency. Some organizations without the resources to maintain on-site mental health teams establish service contracts with off-site service providers who meet with referred clients either at the sheltered or at their facilities. In these situations, a woman's first point of contact with the mental health complex will be her case manager at the shelter, who will then refer her to the on-site or off-site service provider. This experience was Jerusha's, a Nigerian woman who, after telling her case manager that she was hearing voices, was referred to a mental health center, which, she says, "put me in a program" and placed her on "mental ill pills."

Not all shelters have the means to provide comprehensive services, and thus hearing from impoverished women that they had sought out services on their own or were referred for assistance through the other programs they were attending is not unusual (Huey, Fthenos, and Hryniewicz 2012). One means of attempting to access mental health services is by attending a free clinic (medical or mental health). Debra chose this route. While in recovery for a crack cocaine addiction, she felt that something was wrong, so she located a mental health clinic and simply said, "I need help." Her problem, she says, "ended up being depression."

Although many of the women first accessed mental health services only after entering a shelter, others, like Jan and Joanne, had much longer histories as mental health consumers, histories that began prior to becoming homeless. Jan first sought help after the recent death of her mother, which coincided with her involvement in the criminal trial of her ex-husband. Of this period, she says, "I just lost it. I didn't care about living anymore. . . . I was dirty. I stunk. I never got out of bed." Taking the advice of her Alcoholics Anonymous sponsor, Jan sought inpatient treatment at a local hospital. Joanne similarly sought help through self-admission to an inpatient psychiatric hospital when she found herself seriously contemplating jumping in front of a train. Prior to moving to Los Angeles, Grace resided in Las Vegas with an abusive husband. Her first attempts at securing assistance entailed visits to a primary care physician. Sent home with a prescription for alprazolam, she continued in a downward spiral that led to two suicide attempts. The first attempt resulted in Grace being taken into custody when the police found her holed up in her bedroom with a gun. Once deemed sufficiently stable, she was transported by the officers to a psychiatric institution, where she was placed on a seventy-two-hour hold for treatment and observation. This confinement led to a diagnosis of BPD, she reported, but not ongoing therapeutic support. Falling through the cracks in the system, six years later Grace again attempted suicide. Overdosing, she was taken to the emergency room, where "they pumped my stomach and gave me a doctor." Following this episode, she was assigned to psychiatric outpatient services and placed on prescription drugs. Another, Quadra, a victim of both sexual abuse and physical violence, first entered psychiatric treatment through an emergency hospitalization for suicidal threats. Although she had managed to overcome an addiction to crack cocaine in 1992, over the years she continued to struggle with mental health issues, cycling in and out of both homelessness and hospitalizations. Her most recent episode of homelessness began following her release from inpatient treatment for what she describes as "schizophrenia . . . suicidal . . . depression . . . illusions."[2]

One avenue through which a handful of women, such as Suzall, received a diagnosis was as a result of child custody cases with the Department of Children and Family Services (DCFS). As an example, at the time of her interview, Tracee is in the process of trying to block the adoption of her daughter by a foster family. As part of the evaluation process, she was sent for a psychological assessment that resulted in her being diagnosed with PTSD and BPD and placed under the ongoing treatment of a psychiatrist at a local mental health center.

Once women had entered the system, the focus of the clinical examination was typically on an individual's symptomology rather than on her as a whole person with a history that might have some bearing on her present functioning. As previously noted, with the rise of biopsych, such treatment has become fairly standard (Brown 1993). This treatment arises because the subjects of biopsychiatric discourse, as Nikolas Rose has said, have come to "embody or suffer from particular and discrete conditions, which account for behavioral symptoms and pathological conduct . . . each of which is at least a candidate for a unique pathology" (2007, p. 191). Jan's experience of being diagnosed with schizophrenia exemplifies this approach. When asked how she came to receive a diagnosis of schizophrenia, Jan replies: "Whatever interview that I gave him, I answered the questions as honest as I could . . . [and] at that point I didn't see . . . it's just questions they ask you." Connie had been experiencing panic attacks and had located a book on OCD. Armed with information from the book, she sought an appointment with a psychiatrist. She describes the diagnostic process as follows: "The psychiatrist asked, 'What are your symptoms?' So I told her, 'I wash my hands more than once. I'm afraid of death. I get nervous. I get panic.' . . . She said, 'Okay, you have this, this, this. You're going to take this medicine.'" Marybeth describes a similar experience: "It's like, 'How do you feel? Yeah, okay, you got ten minutes. And you're feeling this way because . . .'" Angrily, she adds, "That's not right. It doesn't help get the problem out."

Constructing a Diagnosis

In order to better understand how the power to define women's problems operates, in this section we explore in greater detail a handful of individual stories that illustrate the process by which traumatic distress can become recodified as forms of innate pathology. We are not suggesting that people cannot develop mental illness without trauma, as is clearly not the case. Our focus however is on the role of trauma in the development of mental illness and, most importantly, how trauma need not be ignored in diagnosing and treating mental illness.

Lilly's story represents a case in point. This forty-three-year-old woman grew up in a physically and sexually abusive environment, within which she was passed around to family members because her mother, a drug addict, could not care for her. Lilly left home at fourteen and eventually married. After her marriage, she discovered that her husband was not only actively associated with gangs but physically abusive. She eventually left and, having nowhere to go, found herself in a recurring pattern of homelessness. Her most recent period of homelessness has lasted for the better part of the past twelve years. Of her present situation, she says, "I can say that the twelve years on the streets is better than being with any of my family members . . . [because] the streets were safer for me." Lilly has battled both feelings of depression and episodes of binge drinking. In listening to her words, we discover the predominant theme that comes through is a profound lack of trust in others, which is entirely understandable given the pattern of abuse she has experienced throughout her life. Living on the streets, where she has been sexually assaulted on multiple occasions, has only sharpened her distrust. As a result, she chooses to isolate herself as a form of self-protection. Upon entering psychiatric treatment through her shelter, Lilly's pattern of behavior and distrust of others was awarded the diagnosis of social anxiety disorder, a more recently constructed diagnosis with symptoms that include chronic avoidance of interpersonal contact with strangers and social situations due to fear or anxiety that is disproportional to the actual threat posed by the situation or sociocultural context (APA 2013).[3] Lilly does not feel that her choice to withdraw from others is a form of pathology but an adaptive response to her experiences. She explains,

> They say I have social disease but that's not true . . . it's not that. I'm just smart enough not to have too many people around me because I don't know what they're going to do. I've been in this shit for a long time. I know people. I can look at a person and read them like the back of my hand. I don't want people around me. Not these people.

Maria reported being first diagnosed with BPD at the age of thirteen, when her adoptive family took her to see a psychiatrist because she was exhibiting signs of "acting out." In essence, Maria had begun a persistent pattern of running away. Asked about this diagnosis, she replies, "Oh, the sickness. I was diagnosed with bipolar at a very young age." Her behaviors, however, her "acting out," were clearly linked to the sexual abuse she was experiencing in the home. "My dad sexually abused me a lot," she explains. "My mother pretended like it never happened. To this day she won't admit that it ever happened even though she caught him in the act." Maria's story begins much earlier, though, when she was abandoned at an orphanage in Chile. Her first few years were spent in a foster home in that country before she was adopted at eight by the family within which she experienced the sexual abuse. She left her adoptive home at seventeen, sleeping on friends' sofas and renting hotel rooms. With the exception of a two-year period during which she lived with an abusive partner, she estimates she has been homeless for most of the past fifteen years. She describes a small window of being stably housed as the only time she has had a "permanent place." She has tried to establish herself in a job and home but found it difficult because "I would always go through depressive or angry or whatever moods." Like Lilly, Maria has significant trust issues, which have led her to self-isolate: "I would never let anyone in. I'd never talk to anybody. I was very isolated. I didn't speak to anybody." Marijuana use became a coping tool: "I smoked weed, a lot of weed." Rather than seeing this use as tied to the stresses of life on the streets, she echoes psychiatry by explaining it as "my way of dealing with my mental illness."

Another coping strategy, from which she profited both financially and personally, is shoplifting. Talking about her boosting activities, her voice rises and she says with some pride: "I made a really amazing career out of it." The boosting produces an emotional high that helps her deal with periods of depression. Although she has spent years being told she is bipolar and openly accepts both the diagnosis and the drugs prescribed as the antidote to the chemicals that are said to cause her mood swings, she "keep[s] on forgetting to realize that's an actual sickness." In speaking of her experiences with biopsychiatry and counseling, she forgets again that she has been assigned an illness with a biochemical origin and says of the state of her mental health, "I have things going on with me that are deeply rooted, since I was a baby."

Marybeth is a thirty-nine-year-old African American mother of a twenty-year-old daughter, who estimates that she has been in and out of the mental health system since she was seven years old. Her first exposure to the system came when she was placed in counseling to deal with the effects of severe child abuse. Over the past four years, she and her daughter have bounced from shelter to shelter across the United States, as she struggles to find resources to get back on her feet. She readily admits to not letting go of negative thoughts; however, rather than seeing this behavior as obsessive negative thinking, she sees it as a positive adaptive strategy. She explains, "I'm supposed to think . . . if something's wrong with my life, I'm supposed to get on it, not let it just sit there." Although she has had periods of deep depression, Marybeth views her biggest emotional problem as anger: "Anger is my thing. That's what I'm working on right now. I get completely inflamed." She then proceeds to describe several situations at the shelter where she became "really inflamed." Each of the situations she relates involves incidents where either she or her daughter were patronized or felt disrespected by shelter staff. Reflecting on her situation, we asked if some of her anger is attached to feelings of helplessness over her situation and the environment within which she finds herself. She replies: "It's that, and why am I not being helped after four years? This is what I'm most angry about. I'm trying everything I know. I even got sick in the hospital because I'm doing too much. What do I do? I want to get out of this." Marybeth does not attribute all of her anger to her present circumstances; she acknowledges that some of it is the result of unhealed trauma from her past. "It's because of deeper-rooted reasons," she admits. Over the course of years of mental health treatment, Marybeth's emotional swings, between intense anger and depression, have led to a diagnosis of BPD. At first she accepted this diagnosis as the answer to her emotional distress: "It used to be, 'Something's wrong with you. You're on that bipolar.'" However, reflecting on her moods and how they are clearly linked to significant stressors over the course of her life, she no longer feels this diagnosis is accurate:

> No, I don't [feel I have a chemical imbalance]. [Laughs.] No, I really don't. I feel . . . not to get too deep or anything, but I feel the world has an imbalance, and I'm trying to adjust to it, and they diagnosed me because "you can't get it!" No, I'm not supposed to get this shit! This is fucked up! [Laughs.] I'm sorry, but this is messed up. If you don't have anything wrong with you, or anything going on, and you think this is all right, something's wrong with you. I cried last night. "What is this? Why's this happening?" I said. "I gotta calm down. This is not mine." I get like that and I have to just dissociate. Just focus.

Rachel is a thirty-six-year-old grandmother who grew up with two addicted parents. Rachel herself began using drugs at the age of eleven. In the eighth grade, she stopped going to school and had her first child. This self-described "wild-child running wild" is now homeless for her second time.

She describes herself as "out of balance" and her thoughts as "way off pattern." When asked about the nature of those thoughts, she replies,

> I get confused. I don't know what to do. The voices. Whose was that voice? Was that God's? Was that Jesus's voice? Or was that the devil's voice. So now I'm stuck because I don't know whose voice was who. Most of the time I go with, "That was the devil." Sometimes it could've been God that wanted me to step away or break away from people. I'm thinking, "Why would God not want me to be friends with this person?"

As a result of her feelings of mental confusion and experiences of auditory hallucinations, she was referred to a psychiatrist who provided a diagnosis: "I'm a paranoid schizophrenic." Under psychiatric treatment since 2000, Rachel has also continued to use street drugs, which she believes led her to enter a drug treatment program. She also continues to be plagued by disturbing thoughts and voices that "throw her off every now and then."

Marvella, a fifty-year-old African American woman, grew up in a physically abusive household in Little Rock, Arkansas. She does not say much about it, but she acknowledges that there was also some sexual abuse in her childhood. As an adolescent, she began a pattern of relationships with older men, who were also abusive. By the time she was nineteen, Marvella had already been shot by one former partner. When asked about this event, she reveals this attempt was not the only one made on her life; she carries two sets of scars from separate shootings, which she shows. Tiring of Little Rock, Marvella moved to Denver, where she struggled to hold down a job. Unable to gain a secure footing, she eventually found herself living on the streets of Denver. While living on Colorado streets, she was under constant stress and developed insomnia. Not surprisingly, given the stress and lack of sleep, in time her mental state began to deteriorate: "I found myself walking the streets in the middle of traffic. Because I was in . . . I'm feeling like because of all this conspiracy that's going on in my life, no one's even hitting me. And I'm in traffic. I have my back turned on a one-way street and I don't even know what's coming at me. I was just really stressed out." Marvella had begun to believe that "people were conspiring about me," a belief that came to encompass "the whole city," including the various psychiatrists from whom she sought treatment. Reflecting on her thinking at this time, she summarizes it as "all doctors were in cahoots together." In Denver, she received two different diagnoses: PTSD and schizophrenia. Whereas the PTSD diagnosis recognized the aftereffects of her experiences of extreme physical and sexual victimization, the schizophrenia diagnosis drew on her presentation as someone with auditory hallucinations and paranoid delusions. Of the latter, this woman, who had been living in shelters and on the streets, says, "I felt like people were conspiring about me. I felt like my private life has been invaded. I had no privacy in my life." Referring to her time in Denver, not to discount her diagnosis of schizophrenia, her symptoms were likely exacerbated by factors in her then-present situation, such as the fact that homeless citizens typically lack any privacy or that women commonly report experiences of being abused by trusted friends and acquaintances on the street, problems that can magnify already present symptoms for a traumatized person under chronic stress. Notably, she says that since she has been in Los Angeles, those feelings have diminished substantially: "I feel a sense of peace. Maybe it's because nobody knows me. I don't know anybody. I don't have to worry about my friends trying to backstab me."

Vanessa has been homeless since she was nineteen; she is now forty-four. As a child, she was physically and sexually abused by her biological parents and was taken into foster care at the age of eleven. In one of the foster homes to which she was sent, she experienced sexual abuse from an older adopted son. This abuse led to several attempts at running away, behavior that resulted in Vanessa's placement in a facility for juveniles labeled "hard to place." By the age of twenty, she was addicted to heroin and joined a gang. "I hung out in one area where the drugs are rampant . . . [and] pretty much you didn't sell dope unless you were in the gang, or you pay, you know, what they called taxes, and I wasn't willing to pay those taxes, so I just jumped in, joined." Of this period in her life, she says simply, "I survived." During the time Vanessa has been on the streets, she's been raped and physically assaulted. She has also experienced intimate partner violence, including one episode that resulted in a punctured lung. "My ex-girlfriend stabbed me," she explains. Reflecting on her current state, Vanessa sees herself as having "a lot of . . . um . . . emotional problems" and finds that "with all the baggage of my past, you know, it's still holding me from doing the things that I need to do, like holding down a job, um, even finding a place to live." Vanessa, now in a transitional housing program, is receiving housing assistance; however, she remains traumatized by events in her past. "I still haven't gotten over all the stuff that's happened to me as a child, and I still relive some of that, especially at night." Over the years, she has seen several psychiatrists and received multiple diagnoses. Given her history of trauma, which has manifested in depressed and anxious feelings, as well as in insomnia, that these diagnoses include PTSD, as well as generalized anxiety disorder and major depression, is not surprising. They also include a personality disorder, the name of which Vanessa does not remember, but she kindly offers to go up to her room and bring down a piece of paper that provides the diagnosis. Given Vanessa is a mother with a young child, and it is near that child's bedtime, the offer is politely declined and the discussion moves with Vanessa, a lesbian, offering an explanation for why she believes she was diagnosed with a personality disorder. "They diagnosed me way back when," she says, "you know, they really didn't understand gay and lesbian and transgender. They didn't understand those things. They just thought, 'You know, your personality is just way all over the place.'"

Lindsay was first seen by a psychiatrist at the age of sixteen. Today she is fifty-nine and has been diagnosed as schizophrenic. Her problems started long before her first psychiatric visit, when she was molested by her father as a small child, as well as being physically abused and neglected by both parents. The abuse was discovered and Lindsay was placed in foster care. Later she was sent to live with an aunt. When initially asked what diagnosis she received at sixteen, she does not directly respond: "I have been abused . . . as a child I've been neglected . . . I turned into a toy robot . . . if not, I wouldn't be . . ."[4] Lindsay acknowledges that she has problems managing her emotions, a fact that she attributes, in part, to stress, which increases the volume of the voices she hears: "It's like someone is really wanting me to lose it completely and mentally and not be aware of my own self."

Meredith's story illustrates well how traumatic events can create forms of distress that manifest in thoughts, feelings, and behaviors, which in many cases are interpreted as symptoms of psychological disorders. Meredith is a fifty-six-year-old African American woman who attributes her five years of homelessness to ongoing addictions to crack cocaine and alcohol. Her childhood was spent with a father and two sisters. Although she never reveals whether she too had been molested, she acknowledges that her father sexually abused her sisters for a number of years. One result of this abuse is that Meredith has "a nephew by my dad." She also recalls episodes where she tried to defend her siblings by attempting to beat her father off the younger girls when he was sexually abusing them. While relating these stories, Meredith says of herself, "I've been going mental since I was thirteen." Since then, she has had a string of dysfunctional relationships and a set of addictions she feels helpless to overcome. She also has insomnia and experiences "racing thoughts" and auditory hallucinations. Of the latter, she says, "I hear voices . . . [and] right now I have twelve people I can talk to [in my head] and have a whole conversation." For Meredith, the voices are not terrifying; indeed, when asked whom she might discuss her problems with, she replies that she talks to the voices as a coping strategy. Over the years, Meredith's feelings of depression, coupled with auditory hallucinations, have resulted in diagnoses of BPD and schizophrenia. She signals her acceptance of these diagnoses by how she refers to herself: "I am bipolar, schizophrenic." Despite her adoption of these labels, which come laden with the belief that her brain is chemically malfunctioning, she refers to her present problems as being rooted in untreated trauma. For example, she describes herself as "hurting" from the memories of her childhood. As may be recalled from the last chapter, Meredith struggles with understanding the abuse and overcoming feelings of helplessness. "I try to get it," she admits, "but that overpowering part of what I lived creeps back in there."

The Pastor is a tiny woman, neatly dressed, with a smiling, animated face. Her size and movements remind me immediately of a small, delicate bird. But that appearance belies an enormous energy and enthusiasm that she expends on preaching to the sinners in and around Pasadena's homeless shelters. She would like to be interviewed but first wants to know if the interviewer is Christian. Sensing a possible problem, Laura gives the same answer that she does when unscheduled visitors arrive on her doorstep on Saturday mornings: "We're Jewish." Her smiling face clouds over for a second, and she asks, "What's that?" After a quick explanation, she is smiling again and chatting away happily. Throughout the course of the interview, the Pastor, who is fifty-six, explains how she came to be homeless, what her experiences with various forms of therapeutic and other assistance are, and how she came to be called to her ministry. Her story begins in 1979, as a young woman who was involved in an emotionally and physically abusive relationship with an older man. When the relationship ended, she was "devastated" and fell into a deep depression: "I was really sick." She sought psychiatric assistance at that time and was placed on diazepam but ultimately lost her job and her home. She then decided to restart her life by moving back home with her mother. For the next twenty-two years, she remained with her mother, never marrying or having children. When her mother died in 2002, followed by her brother, the Pastor says of herself, "My whole life was gone." She again fell into a deep depression, during which she became "really suicidal." In 2007, the Pastor became homeless and began making the rounds of various shelters, looking for help and places to stay. She says of the time, "My thoughts became wrong. I became unsound. I allowed myself to be in shelter, shelter, shelter, and they never really helped me, and I didn't help myself, right." Clarifying what she means by her mind becoming "unsound," she again refers to a pattern of suicidal thinking. In order to "help herself in the right way," the Pastor, as is the case with many of the destitute women residing in and around shelters, turned to religious belief as a form of guidance and solace. The content of her beliefs, however, put her at distinct odds with the views of her shelter case manager and the mental health practitioners she was sent to see: she wanted to eschew a medicated approach to managing her depression in favor of scripture and prayer. These views were hardened after she had a bad reaction to the drug quetiapine, classified as an atypical antipsychotic drug. "If it's not from God," she says, "I don't want it." In clinical parlance, the Pastor is exhibiting signs of "hyperreligiosity," often associated with schizophrenia and other delusional disorders (Brewerton 1994). Although we are not questioning the validity of the Pastor's diagnosis, we do note that her case is not uniquely exceptional in terms of the content of her religious beliefs: exposure to the wide range of forms of Christian thought and practice in the United States and elsewhere easily demonstrates this point. Thus, the fact that the Pastor's chosen solution to her problems can be interpreted as a sign of a delusional disorder reflects a wider problem in the diagnosis and treatment of the problems of black women in the United States. Specifically, for those who come from evangelical sects, a dependence on God that would be seen as very normal in those sects might be seen as hyperreligiosity by someone unfamiliar with the specific subculture. This fact was brought home when a former member of the research team, herself raised in such a background, had a conversation with a woman about how Satan uses people to hurt others. Rather than dismissing or challenging what might be seen by some as an irrational belief, the team member entered into a discussion of relevant scriptures. That woman, along with a disproportionate number of largely impoverished, black citizens in the United States, was diagnosed as schizophrenic (Bresnahan et al. 2007; Eack et al. 2012; Pavokov, Lewis, and Lyons 1989; Perry, Neltner, and Allen 2013; Snowden 2003), which raises an interesting question of the extent to which hyperreligiosity may factor in the creation of biopsychiatric diagnoses when the patient and doctor do not share a common worldview, despite the intention in the DSM to control for such situations (APA 2013). In the case of the Pastor, her adoption of this particular worldview has allowed her to make peace with her situation and see it as a means of sustaining a calling that brings her joy. Thus, when leaving the shelter, we were not at all surprised to find the Pastor quietly standing outside its gates, with her self-printed brochures in hand, waving while she waits for someone in spiritual need to walk by.

I Am. I Have. I Don't.

When a diagnostic label is applied to a collection of symptoms, it can serve to structure the psychiatrist's understanding of an individual's problems and therefore become a tool to set a course of treatment. However, it may also be used by various institutions (i.e., the shelter, the prison) to understand, respond, and control individuals and their behavior. Further, and most importantly for the purpose of gaining insight into how biopsychiatric power manifests, individuals may use their diagnoses to make sense of their own thoughts, feelings, and behaviors, and to serve as an identity by which they come to represent themselves to others. Conversely, diagnoses, and the labels to which they are attached, can also be rejected in whole or in part by their recipients. Thus, of the forms of biopsychiatric power enumerated here, the power of diagnosis is perhaps the one that affords an individual the greatest opportunity to exercise a degree of choice (of course, prescribed treatment can be forced on an individual in select circumstances). In this section, we examine the means by which diagnoses are variously accepted or rejected by the women interviewed for this project and the reasons they articulate for the choices they made.[5]

Analyses of the statements made by women who accepted the diagnoses they received reveal two primary forms through which this acceptance is signaled. The first is through words that indicate the diagnosis is viewed as an identity to which the interviewee willingly ascribed. This expression of acceptance was typically found in statements containing the words *I am* or *I'm*, as in "I am bipolar." Examples have already been provided by both Rachel and Meredith, who refer to themselves as "a paranoid schizophrenic" and a "bipolar, schizophrenic," respectively. There is also Kathy, who had been diagnosed with BPD and PTSD and has openly adopted her diagnoses as identity labels, particularly the bipolar label. She admits that this was not always the case: "When they first told me I felt like, 'Oh my God, I'm stigmatized. I'm mentally ill!'" Today, though, she refers to herself as bipolar and talks frequently, without prompting, about how "being bipolar" has affected her:

> You feel such a barrage of feelings. Right now I know I spider everywhere. It's like a web. I jump and jump and jump because I have trouble staying focused . . . [and] I'm used to talking in my head. I have a constant negative dialogue in my head. Now it's like *boom, boom, boom.* My neurons fire off. I'll be here, there, and everywhere. . . .
>
> It's like chronic depression. It feels like I want to sleep. I don't want to participate. Yes, I become very antisocial. I don't want to be out. I don't want to take care of myself. It's like someone just sucked the life out of me. I don't know if you've ever heard of this before, but bipolars love their mania. They love their upside. You feel like, "Dang! I'm so productive." You feel so euphoric and energetic. It's almost like an addiction. It reminds me of when I was on speed. I love it.

Kathy not only accepts her bipolar diagnosis as an identity but also believes that her problems are caused by a chemical imbalance. In discussing this acceptance, Kathy acknowledges that doing so has a certain social utility:

self-describing as bipolar gives her a way to explain her present problems to others without having to invoke her past. She is left without having to reveal she was pregnant at fourteen years old and living on the streets of Los Angeles. "I learned that [in telling the story] you just retraumatize yourself again. It's like it's happening all over again . . . [so] I try to stay super official and not go into detail." Of her ability to simply say, "I'm bipolar," she says, "Thank God for labels." In this regard Kathy is not dissimilar from Freda, who used the opportunity of her diagnosis to go back to school and take college psychology courses in order to develop insight into her thoughts and behaviors. Among other things she learned was mindful awareness techniques and the art of "self-talk" in order to address problematic thoughts.

Other women who self-identify using a diagnostic label include Kim, who grew up in foster care and has since been the victim of both intimate partner violence and sexual assault. When asked if she has experienced any feelings of anxiety or depression, she bypasses the question, instead referring to herself with a clinical label: "I'm bipolar." Teneka was sexually assaulted by multiple men, including family members, and later victimized by an abusive partner. When similarly asked if she has experienced any periods of anxiety or depression, she replies, "Me, I'm what you call a managed depression person."

The second way acceptance of a diagnosis is typically signaled is through an individual describing herself as "having" a mental illness. For example, Marcia is a fifty-year-old woman who had, until she entered a shelter, been living with what she describes as an overbearing, controlling mother. Referring to the feelings she has been bottling up, she says she would like to be able to say, "Mom, let me go. Let me go. Fifty years old, c'mon." Marcia, who is actively looking for employment, has been hiding the fact that she moved into a shelter from her mother. She reveals she would rather live in the shelter than continue to live with what she feels is emotional abuse. "Her pressures get enough," Marcia explains. Despite her depression beginning before she entered homelessness, summing up where she is mentally and emotionally, Marcia does not define herself during the interview as someone dealing with low self-esteem and an overbearing mother. Instead, she self-describes as someone who has "got depression" and "[has] mental issues." Ella, as may be recalled from the previous chapter, has survived homelessness for about four years by living, off and on, under a freeway. She was sexually abused as a child, was physically and sexually assaulted multiple times on the streets, and, as noted in the previous chapter, was once left for dead by the side of a road. When asked about the nature of the problems she faces, she does not describe herself as a trauma survivor but as someone who "has" a schizoaffective disorder.

Notably, whether consciously or not, several of the women who accepted their diagnoses self-described in terms or phrases that echoed biopsych discourse. They internalized their diagnoses and the associated stigma and master status. Callie provides a small example of this when asked why she was placed on the drug quetiapine: "Just because my nerves, my paranoia, my unstableness, my forgetfulness. Just a decline in my whole presentation." Although Zakiah has been homeless off and on for the past four years, instead of attributing her low moods to her present situation or to past experiences of growing up with a "mentally unstable" mother, domestic violence, or sexual assault, she invokes biopsych discourse and her stigma in describing herself as "clinically depressed." Similarly, in speaking of depression, she attributes her low moods to chemical imbalances in her brain.

Perhaps the most notable example of evidence of biopsych speak in the words of an interviewee came from Grace. Grace has experienced a lot of emotional and physical pain. She was sexually assaulted as a teenager: "I got raped at sixteen by five guys," she tells. Later, she entered a highly abusive relationship with a man who beat her and brought other women into their home. Grace became dependent on alcohol and crack cocaine and spent some time in jail. In describing the nature of the issues she has faced, Grace does not refer to this past. Instead, she says of herself, "I have depression. I have manic depressive." Like Kathy, Grace embraced her diagnosis as offering a preferable answer as to why her life had been in a state of chaos. "I thought I was crazy," she says, "so for six years I stayed locked in my house." Now she sees herself not as "crazy," but as having a condition: "I've got a chemical imbalance." When asked about the nature of this imbalance, she promptly replies, "My serotonin and my norepinephrine aren't balanced." For some women, such as Mercy, who has been diagnosed with depression, acceptance of the biopsych worldview comes with a harsh reality that she struggles to digest: "What I have can't be fixed, they think."

Not all diagnoses, or the labels they come attached with, are readily or otherwise accepted. As we saw with Vanessa, some women feel that the diagnoses they received were in error, the result of faulty assumptions or misunderstandings. Such was also the case with Jan, who had been diagnosed as paranoid schizophrenic. She received this diagnosis the first time she checked herself into inpatient psychiatric treatment. She believes that the staff at the psychiatric unit she had committed herself to were "people that don't care" and that the hospital itself had a financial incentive for giving her this diagnostic label: "The higher diagnosis they give you, the worse diagnosis they give you, the more money they make. It's all about that dolla'." Rather than seeing herself as a paranoid schizophrenic, or as having schizophrenia, she feels that she has been living through a period of major depression.

In other cases, the rejection of a diagnosis was more subtle. For example, in speaking of herself and her problems, a woman might emphasize one aspect of a diagnosis, thus downplaying what she perceived to be diagnoses she either disagreed with or found more stigmatizing. Toni, who grew up with a stepfather who molested children and beat her mother in front of them, self-describes as "I'm depressed." In fact, she made this statement several times in the interview. However, when asked what diagnoses she had received from the psychiatrist she was seeing, she replies, "They just diagnosed me as a manic depressant with psychotic features." Similarly, in reference to herself, Tracee says, "I have PTSD." Later in the interview, when she is discussing what she sees as the failure of DCFS to protect her child, she reveals in her anger another diagnosis that she had chosen to conceal. Referring to both her DCFS social worker and her psychiatrist, she says, "They want to call me bipolar and all that? I'm gonna show them."

Trauma: An Obscure Phenomenon?

The purpose of diagnosis is ostensibly to identify the nature and cause of a condition in order to select the most appropriate method of treatment. Thus, one might say that the practice of diagnosis is revelatory. However, as the preceding pages make evident, in relation to the emotional, behavioral, cognitive, social, and other problems experienced by homeless women, the diagnostic process is seen to obscure as much as it may illuminate.

In essence, biopsych and some of its practitioners treat trauma as a largely obscure—that is, less important—phenomenon. Either they do so in clinical examinations or they act in ways that leave patients feeling that their lived experiences, their histories, are deemed irrelevant to the matter of who they are and how they function. Thus they render what is felt to be diagnostic judgments that attribute fault to women's brains rather than the interpersonal and social conditions that create suffering, and, if they do focus on trauma, they do so in ways that are not fully appreciated by the women. Thus, the signs of distress exhibited by girls and women who have been sexually abused seem to be reduced to their unstable moods (specifically being "bipolar"), as we saw in the cases of Maria and Tracee. Further, extreme stress, coupled with the effects of untreated trauma, seems unaccounted for in the mental confusion, delusional thinking, and hallucinations these women experience. Marvella's "geographical cure" is therefore not evidence of what can happen when such stress is removed; it is reduced to being simply coincidental that her purported chemical imbalance righted itself when she removed herself from a highly adverse situation. No matter what her diagnosis, and symptoms, acknowledgment of her trauma in a way that she understands and can use to understand her own situation and feelings is missing in her story. This conclusion begs the question, acknowledged or not, that plagues the practice: How does one explain when depression or any episode of mental illness ends? With or without intervention, each will eventually cease but when is never known. It's almost as though mental health has its own terms and conditions.

As such, when patient history is deemed, well, less relevant to the process of diagnosis, and trauma removed from full consideration of causes and effects, concerns must be raised about the potential for both misdiagnosis or overdiagnosis. Further, although both phenomena can happen to male psychiatric patients, history reveals that women have borne much of the brunt of sexist assumptions in diagnosis, both in the creation of diagnostic categories and in their application (Chesler 2005; Chrisler and Caplan 2002). As a result, women's emotional problems have been more frequently treated as evidence of individual psychopathology, and clinicians have been more willing to affix harmful diagnostic labels upon female patients (Chesler 2005). In the case of homeless women in the United States, a host of sociodemographic factors can compound to further increase the complexity of diagnostic processes, which leaves a higher margin for diagnostic errors. These factors include realities like the fact that homeless women are impoverished, many are African American or from other racial and ethnic minority groups, and some come from minority cultural or religious backgrounds. Thus, diagnostic and therapeutic models based on conformity to middle-class, white standards of belief and behavior dominant in the United States will necessarily, albeit unintentionally, pathologize those who do not conform (Bullock 2004). This conclusion is not simply conjecture; a raft of studies demonstrate evidence of the impact on mental health of gender bias (Becker and Lamb 1994; Ford and Widiger 1989; Lindsay, Sankis, and Widiger 2000; Widiger 1998), racial bias (Arroyo 1996; Bell, Williamson, and Chien 2008; Pavkov, Lewis, and Lyons 1989; Perry, Neltner, and Allen 2013), and socioeconomic bias (Bullock 2004; Lutfey 2013; Routh and King 1972), and as a result, we can safely say that being an impoverished woman of color increases one's odds of being diagnosed with a chronic, stigmatizing disorder.

The phenomenon of multiple diagnoses was also all too common among the homeless women interviewed. Although a handful of the women received more than one diagnosis from the same clinician, usually with anxiety disorders and depression seen as comorbid conditions, others, which represents a rather concerning fact, received multiple diagnoses as a result of having seen several clinicians over years of treatment. This fact evinces the temporal component of symptoms as well as the challenge of working with the human brain. Marvella is a case in point: she has been variously told she has PTSD and schizophrenia, two very different conditions, with different ascribed causes, treatment modalities, and prognoses. Marvella's example perfectly highlights the variability in clinical approaches and clinician judgments and the net diagnostic effects of these differences. At one point, her condition was likely assessed in light of her history as a domestic violence survivor, and, later, another specialist seemed to focus predominantly, if not exclusively, on her symptoms. Thus, two different psychiatrists arrived at two separate and very different judgments. Her example also reveals something else: when two clinicians were presented with the same person, in this instance an impoverished African American woman, the one who saw her in light of her symptoms also ascribed her behaviors to an innate pathological condition, a highly stigmatized condition.

Although the women's stories clearly indicate that some clinicians do fail to appropriately consider the role that trauma plays in shaping the issues facing the vast majority of women who participated in this study, the stories also make evident that not all of the women saw themselves or their present situations as signs of biological malfunctioning. Certainly, some, such as Grace and Kathy, did refer to themselves as struggling with a biochemical imbalance. However, others, notably Vanessa and Meredith, adopted some or all of the diagnostic labels clinicians have affixed to them, even though their own views of the causes of their problems contradicted the biochemical explanations that come with those labels. How, then, can the adoption of such labels by individuals whose beliefs contradicted the assumptions that come with these labels be explained?

One way to explain this apparent form of cognitive dissonance is to suggest that such individuals simply lack awareness of the meaning of those labels or see them as sufficiently fluid or permeable as to include emotional or psychological states generated by environmental causes. Although the latter may be the case for some of the women, such as those diagnosed solely with major depression, the same cannot be said for women diagnosed with those conditions exclusively attributed to biological causes. Also, contending they simply lack knowledge or understanding is not only unduly dismissive but also not supported by this study. Of course, there is another way of looking at this issue, and that is to see it as an effect of biopsychiatric power, exacerbated by structural violence and stigma. As detailed in Chapter 2, all three are dominant forces—culturally, socially, and economically—within contemporary societies. Each is tied to labels, of which psychiatry's are imbued with the pronounced authority of "science." An additional power dimension emerges when one also considers the unequal social locations of homeless women versus clinicians, as well as their respective roles in the therapeutic process. The former are troubled, often desperate women with few alternate resources, whereas the latter are the accredited experts whose job is to render diagnostic judgments. The clinicians' judgments not only are authoritative but are backed by cultural support and the weight of mainstream social norms. We are not suggesting that women cannot resist such judgments. We have seen they can and they do. We rather are suggesting that a diagnosis carries enough social weight that it can render resistance a more difficult task, particularly when almost all of these women are individuals who are desperate for solutions that hold the promise of lifting them out of their present circumstances.

The act of diagnosis is, in and of itself, clearly a powerful one. However, although diagnosis serves to identify both a condition and its perceived underlying causes, it is often undertaken as a prelude to what can be understood as another manifestation of biopsychiatric power: prescription.

Notes

1. Worth noting is that individuals who are not using a shelter—that is, they are sleeping rough and may be unwilling for a variety of reasons to use homelessness-related services—are targeted by community outreach workers, who will attempt to link them back into medical, mental health, and other services, usually with varying degrees of success. As the interviews were conducted through homeless shelters, none of the women in this study were sleeping rough at the time of her interview; however, prior to entering a shelter, several, such as Ella, had been sleeping rough for extended periods of time.

2. A recurring theme within the histories of several of the women who had been admitted to inpatient treatment was the loss of their housing. At least half a dozen women told Laura directly that, upon release, their rental units were no longer available to them. Freda is one: "I ended up homeless because I was in the hospital for twenty days. I lost my job. I lost my apartment. I had to drop out of school." Mercy is another. When asked a question about the "side effects" of the drugs she is presently taking, she joked, "Yeah, you get out of the hospital, [and] you become homeless."

3. Social anxiety disorder replaced social phobia in the DSM-V (APA 2013).

4. This passage is verbatim. Lindsay's halting speech pattern is perhaps the result of a condition called alogia (see the introductory section of Chapter 5 for more information on this condition).

5. For insight into the "presentation of homelessness," see Snow and Anderson (1993).

5

Prescriptions for an "Improved Life"

Carly is one of those individuals who enters a room and you feel that a bright ball of energy has descended upon you. She's tough, smart, and wickedly funny and an accomplished street hustler. She makes money selling chilled water on the streets of Los Angeles and on the city's metro lines. Although she's clearly adept at the basic laws of capitalism, proudly undercutting and outselling her competitors, she reveals a softer side when telling a story of giving water away to a hot and thirsty child whose parents did not have the money for a bottle. In listening to her stories, it's clear that she has managed to survive on the strength of her wits and personality, first in a series of foster homes and then as a youth living on the streets. Today, at thirty-seven, she's residing in a shelter, and not for the first time, despite the fact, as she says, "I don't really do too much the shelter thing. I don't really do Skid Row at all."

When Carly was asked if she had ever been incarcerated, she tells of being sent to county jail for unpaid transit tickets, an experience she describes as "kind of like a rape of your freedom." Her next words are chilling: "You get raped inside too. Literally, physically." Then she relates the following experience:

> One day I was in the thing and I heard somebody crying out for help. And you're in a fucking box. A brick box. So I was like . . . I couldn't do anything. I couldn't see . . . [and] unfortunately, that's one of my setbacks, [that] I'm always trying to help somebody. . . . Come to find it was a mentally ill lady, who really wasn't capable of taking care of herself, getting raped. She was five months pregnant and in custody seven. Right here in [location removed]. I was just in for an MTA [Metro Transit Authority] ticket.

Carly, who has survived physical and sexual assault in childhood and as an adult, was left feeling emotionally raw from this experience. As she speaks of it, the aftereffects are obvious: she is visibly angry, her voice rising, her hands moving. She volunteers what happened next in a tight voice. She went to see the jail doctor because the experience had left her unable to sleep. Already on antidepressants for major depression, she reports that the doctor's response was to prescribe drugs that would, in effect, sedate her further. "When I told the doctor [what had happened]," she says, "they gave me more medication . . . they gave me more medication to put me to sleep more." She laughs bitterly and adds, "That didn't really work out too well." Not only was the drug she was given to treat her "condition" ineffective in suppressing her feelings at the time of the incident, but it also had no impact on the rage and pain she continues to carry with her. Involved in an altercation recently with the police where she says she was "attacked" by officers, she became incensed over what she saw as another failure of "the system" in its attempt to "be protecting and serving." As a result, she fought back. Describing the situation, she says, "I was laughing at them while they were kicking my ass. They're like, 'This bitch is crazy.'" She simply shrugs, "I'm like, 'Whatever.'"

The second manifestation of psychiatric power in homeless communities is found in the power to prescribe; that is, having defined the individual's condition, the doctor establishes the mode and course of its treatment. Within the biopsych worldview, we take issue when treatment comes primarily in one form: neurochemical regulators. These regulators are used to suppress positive symptoms of the biological disorders said to be underlying women's "abnormal" thoughts, feelings, and behaviors.[1] Thus, in essence, the power to prescribe is really the ability to control individual behaviors, thoughts, and feelings through suppression. Women are told, as too often has been the case over history, that the suppression of these thoughts and behaviors is for "their own good" (Ehrenreich and English 2005), and this belief is variously accepted or rejected based on individual responses to the drugs used and the extent to which those responses are received as positive and beneficial by the individual patient, the clinician, and the institutions that structure her life.

The focus of this chapter is on the former, the individual and the types of psychiatric drugs she has been prescribed and how she perceives and experiences their use. We begin by looking first at the types of drugs women have been prescribed before turning to the issue of therapy and the extent to which psychiatric drugs are employed as the sole therapeutic intervention. Then we examine the issue of drug effects, revealing first that, for some women, drugs are seen as providing beneficial effects, which we do not discount. These effects are typically described in terms of either symptom abatement or as a leveling effect that is said to allow women the opportunity to engage in regimens of self-care and self-improvement. However, with a closer analysis of the statements of women in this group, we find that, for many, the primary benefit received is often one of sedation. The sedative effects of many of these drugs allow individuals to better tolerate both the symptoms of the trauma they experience, as well as the miseries associated with their present circumstances. In exploring the provision of such drugs, we also consider the stories of women who either had experienced no noticeable improvement from their use or had noted adverse effects. The latter leads to a discussion of what providers term as "resistance" and the reasons women give for being treatment noncompliant. Finally, we turn to the issue of improvement and the extent to which women believe that psychiatric drugs contribute to improvements in their lives.

Pills

As noted in Chapter 3, the drugs women were prescribed typically fell into four broad classes: antidepressants, anxiolytics, mood stabilizers, and antipsychotics. Of these, antidepressants were the most frequently prescribed. They were prescribed not only for individuals diagnosed with depression but for those who wanted to manage symptoms associated with anxiety and the depressive phases of BPD. Carole takes the commonly prescribed drug sertraline (an SSRI) in hope of managing the symptoms of major depression. Michelle, who recently gave up custody of her children, is also taking sertraline for depression and panic attacks. A number of the women who have been diagnosed as schizophrenic were also prescribed one of the newer-generation antidepressants. Jan, who has been diagnosed as schizophrenic reportedly as a result of her experience of persecutory beliefs, had been prescribed the antidepressant fluoxetine (an SSRI) and the antipsychotic drug quetiapine. Melissa, who experiences auditory hallucinations, is on fluoxetine, among other drugs. Women with PTSD were also prescribed antidepressants. Tracee has been diagnosed with both PTSD and BPD and is taking the SSRI escitalopram, as well as the heavily sedating drug trazodone (a tetracyclic antidepressant). Marvella is also on escitalopram for symptoms that have been variously diagnosed as belonging to the conditions of PTSD and schizophrenia.

Most of the women diagnosed with anxiety disorders have also been prescribed antidepressants, with only three exceptions. One was Kesha, whose bouts of hormone-related anxiety, diagnosed as "borderline OCD," she tells Laura, led to, first, a prescription for the ADHD drug atomoxetine and then to a prescription for sertraline. Joelle is another exception. Despite the fact she was a known drug dealer and addict, Joelle was first given the benzodiazepine alprazolam. Then she was withdrawn from this drug "because they said it was addictive." Joelle is now on the drug aripiprazole, an atypical antipsychotic typically used to treat schizophrenia.

Several of the women had been diagnosed as having BPD and yet few were prescribed mood stabilizers. More frequently, they received prescriptions for drugs categorized as antidepressants or as antipsychotics. One of the few exceptions was Renee, who had been treated with lithium. Marybeth, similarly diagnosed as bipolar, was on a newer drug lamotrigine,[2] as was Alex. Rachel, who has been diagnosed as schizophrenic, has also been prescribed lamotrigine.

After antidepressants, the second most frequently prescribed class of psychiatric drugs were antipsychotics. These drugs were prescribed to treat not only delusional disorders but also a range of symptoms linked to major depression and BPD. When asked, women were most likely to say they had been prescribed either quetiapine or aripiprazole (both atypical antipsychotics). For example, among the psychiatric drugs Tess was prescribed while incarcerated was quetiapine. Joelle had also been prescribed quetiapine. Tracee was prescribed aripiprazole, as was Candace. Jan, whose most recent prescription was for fluoxetine, is one of the few women who had been exposed to both the older and newer antipsychotic drugs: while hospitalized for inpatient treatment, Jan had been administered both quetiapine and chlorpromazine.[3] Some of the women had also been prescribed risperidone.[4] Alex, for instance, was taking risperidone along with lamotrigine, as was Hannah, whose psychiatrist had paired the drug with the older antipsychotic drug perphenazine (a phenothiazine).

A notable theme in several of the women's discussions of the psychiatric drug prescriptions they had received was the issue of polypharmacy, referring to the use of four or more medications by one person. A number of them were taking multiple prescribed drugs, often to manage what were perceived to be the symptoms of multiple psychiatric diagnoses. Tracee represents a case in point: she is on the sedative trazodone, the antipsychotic aripiprazole, and the antidepressant escitalopram for PTSD and BPDs. Nicole had recently been diagnosed with both PTSD and a seizure disorder and was taking both the antiepileptic drug levetiracetam as well as two psychiatric drugs, olanzapine (an atypical antipsychotic drug) and lithium. Other women were on multiple drugs simply to manage multiple symptoms. For example, Melissa was on fluoxetine for feelings of depression and some other unnamed drug in order to help her sleep. Rachel was not only on lamotrigine, one of the drugs deemed a mood stabilizer, but also on fluoxetine, a so-called mood elevator, and quetiapine, an antipsychotic with sedating effects. Angelique, who had been diagnosed as schizophrenic and has an extensive history of cycling in and out of psychiatric facilities and jails, was on four different drugs: citalopram, quetiapine, clonazepam, and trazodone. During her recitation of drugs she has been prescribed over the years, Angelique notes that the number of drugs she is presently on was reduced following an incident during which she passed out in front of a nurse after taking her prescriptions. Kelly is also on a cocktail of psychiatric drugs that includes lorazepam, citalopram, bupropion, and trazodone. When queried about her lorazepam dosage,[5] she replies, "I take one in the morning, one at bed, and however many I need during the day."

Other women were dealing with not only mental health issues but also a range of health conditions. Elise, age fifty-four, had been diagnosed as schizophrenic, was dealing with high blood pressure, and had recently been diagnosed as having a tumor on her liver. Aside from the blood pressure drugs and other prescriptions she was taking, she had also been prescribed a regimen that included citalopram, quetiapine, and clozapine. When Bobbie, who has been diagnosed as having schizophrenia and severe depression, is asked what she has been prescribed, she begins pulling bottles out of her bag: "I'm on a lot, not just psych meds, physical and mental. Risperdal, I take two milligrams. Then I'm on Zoloft, and I'm on trazodone. Benadryl for anxiety. I take other meds for diabetes and high blood pressure."

Some women were on so many drugs—psychiatric, pain, blood pressure, and diabetes medication and other pharmaceuticals for various health conditions—that they carried with them a list of drugs, dosages, and instructions as to when to take each pill. Amy is a case in point: when asked what prescriptions she had received in response to her diagnoses of PTSD and depression, she thinks for a moment and then replies, "I'm taking Risperdal," before stopping to take out a list from her purse. Reading the list, she says, "I have Risperdal. I have trazodone and Zoloft." When I ask Lee, who is struggling with severe depression and suicidal ideations, if she has any significant illnesses, she replies:

> LEE: You wanna know what I got? I got so many prescriptions I just went and got the paper [see Photo 5.1]. I have diabetes. I have high blood pressure. I have pulmonary hypertension and a mood disorder.
>
> LAURA: You've got eight different prescriptions.
>
> LEE: I know. That's why I went and got the paper. . . . And I don't take that [lorazepam] much. It's just a point-five, but it helps.
>
> LAURA: Do you take it every day or just when you feel stressed?

LEE: My therapist has me doing it every day to keep it continual, so that it's not when I need it. I take one in the morning and one in the evening. It just keeps me regulated, so I don't have to take it every time I get upset.

LAURA: How long have you been on the lorazepam for?

LEE: Since about February.

This interview with Lee took place in late May of the same year. Lee is saying that for about three months her psychiatrist has had her taking a highly addictive drug, a benzodiazepine that works by producing a calming, sedative effect on the user, twice daily rather than occasionally, "as needed." With daily use, Lee's potential for addiction clearly increases.

Elsewhere, Laura Huey and colleagues (2012) document the problem of physicians and mental health workers diagnosing individuals while they are actively using street drugs, which can have a significant impact on their thoughts, feelings, and behaviors. Of equal seriousness are physicians prescribing psychotropic drugs to individuals who may be using crystal meth, crack, or other drugs that similarly cross the blood-brain barrier and who are therefore already experiencing impaired cognition, emotion, behavior, motor function, and so on. This worry is not an idle one: several of the women in this study, such as Rachel (discussed in Chapter 4) and Kerry (discussed later in this chapter), are actively using street drugs while also

Photo 5.1 Lee's List of Prescriptions, Los Angeles

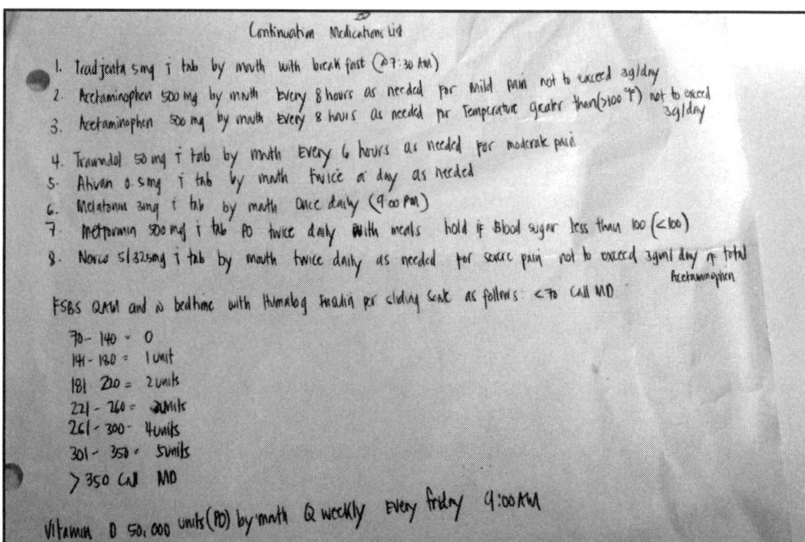
Continuation Medications list

1. Tradjenta 5mg i tab by mouth with breakfast (@7:30 AM)
2. Acetaminophen 500 mg by mouth every 8 hours as needed for mild pain not to exceed 3g/day
3. Acetaminophen 500 mg by mouth every 8 hours as needed for Temperature greater than (>100 °F) not to exceed 3g/day
4. Tramadol 50 mg i tab by mouth every 6 hours as needed for moderate pain
5. Ativan 0.5mg i tab by mouth twice a day as needed
6. Melatonin 3mg i tab by mouth once daily (9:00 PM)
7. Metformin 500 mg i tab PO twice daily with meals hold if Blood sugar less than 100 (<100)
8. Norco 5/325mg i tab by mouth twice daily as needed for severe pain not to exceed 3gm/day of total Acetaminophen

FSBS QAM and @ bedtime with Humalog Insulin per sliding scale as follows: <70 call MD

70 - 140 = 0
141 - 180 = 1 unit
181 - 220 = 2 units
221 - 260 = 3 units
261 - 300 = 4 units
301 - 350 = 5 units
>350 call MD

Vitamin D 50,000 units (PO) by mouth Q weekly Every friday 9:00 AM taking prescribed pharmaceuticals, with the potential for very serious adverse health effects and other consequences.

A final issue raised during an inventory of women's prescription histories is the fact that some had very long histories with biopsychiatry and prescription drugs. Freda, who is only thirty-two, has been placed on several different drugs already in order to treat the symptoms of her bipolar diagnosis. She lists them for me: "Zyprexa, Neurontin, Seroquel, Risperdal. I've been on . . . I didn't take the lithium because it's too many side effects. Right now I'm on Abilify." Elise's journey through biopsychiatry began in Tennessee in the 1970s. Sexually assaulted as a young teenager, her world fell apart and she was subsequently diagnosed as schizophrenic at the age of sixteen. The forms of psychiatric treatment Elise has received have included the drugs thioridazine, trifluoperazine, and fluphenazine, as well as electroshock therapy. As stated previously, she is presently on three psychiatric drugs and says of them, "It's hard for me to take psych meds because I have been on so many of them."

Just Drugs?

One issue we sought to explore was the extent women who had been prescribed psychiatric drugs were also receiving some form of therapy, whether from a psychiatrist, psychologist, or other mental health worker. The responses received varied depending on where a woman was residing. Those staying at one of the better-funded shelters were typically provided access to a psychiatrist as well as to on-site counseling services with licensed clinical therapists. Others were residing in shelters that provide off-site services through nearby mental health groups, usually staffed with therapists and social workers. Of course, those who had been sleeping rough had greater difficulties accessing services, as did women staying in shelters with far fewer resources upon which to draw. In some instances, access to counseling services varied based on the type of program to which a woman had been assigned at her shelter. Those placed in a designated mental health program were provided greater access to both a psychiatrist and a range of counseling services. Those whose problems were not viewed as the result of a mental illness by their case manager were not placed in such programs and, as noted in the previous chapter, instead sought assistance on their own initiative through primary care physicians or mental health clinics.

At previous shelters Melissa could not access therapy because there was "no funding, the money's not there." She is now more fortunate because her present shelter has a mental health team that includes a psychiatrist, counselors, and therapy-oriented groups and workshops. She is on a regimen of fluoxetine and an unnamed sleeping pill, and, until her appointments "got messed up," was also receiving one-on-one sessions with a counselor. Like Melissa, most women receiving both counseling and psychiatric drugs see a therapist for the former and a psychiatrist for the latter. This division of labor is exemplified in a statement made by Maria, who says she "got hooked up with this amazing place" where she gets "seen once a month by the medication doctor to make sure that the medication's working right. And I get to see a therapist once a week." Lee is also in this group: "I see a therapist to talk about my problems, issues, [and] then I have a psychiatrist who I get my medication from." So too is Cora, who credits the staff at her mental health center with helping her learn "how to deal with the changes, to roll with it." She adds, "If it wasn't for my mental health people, I don't think I would've made it. They're the people I can ask, tell them no holds barred, exactly what's going on." Toni, an Inuit woman who is on antidepressants, sees her psychiatrist every two weeks and a therapist on a weekly basis. She feels fortunate because she can talk to both about "the past and whatever goes on during the week." In speaking with Alex, we learn she has been introduced to trauma-informed therapy, an approach that recognizes that underlying trauma can create the distress often seen in individuals' lives. Alex repeatedly references her history of sexual abuse and rape as her "trauma." When asked if she has had therapeutic counseling focused on trauma, she replies, "Yes, in the classes and in speaking about it with the psychologist." As part of her therapeutic experience, Alex is actively involved in learning tools for managing her symptoms, doing homework assignments to help her grow through the process, and reading up on her conditions. She is asked if she finds this process empowering, to which she responds, "I want to know about me and see that if this does happen to me, it's okay. I can feel an emotion. I can read and feel sentimental and cry. Or I can feel angry and I say, 'It's okay; it's a process." Principally, what Alex, in her words, has learned about herself through this process is that feeling her emotions is "okay" and that her anger and despair are "normal" for someone who is a trauma survivor.

Alex is fortunate: many of the women interviewed for this project are not receiving comprehensive counseling and are, instead, only seeing a psychiatrist or primary care physician and thus receiving only psychiatric drugs. For instance, Joelle had previously been seeing a psychologist, but, since her release from prison, her only contact with the mental health system is through a psychiatrist. Of these visits, she says, "She gave me medication and that's what they do." Fifty-nine-year-old Vera is taking fluoxetine for major depression. She describes her visits to the psychiatrist very simply:

"We talk about meds." When asked for clarification about the nature of these appointments, she explains, "That is where there is [a] difference between a psychologist and a psychiatrist. Psychiatrists don't talk." Sheila's psychiatrist speaks, but it's to find out "how it's going. Is the medication . . . do I feel a difference? Am I able to sleep? Do I have flashbacks?" Sheila's psychiatrist also offers advice on how to manage the PTSD and major depression she has been diagnosed with: "'Get out and don't stay in.' Sometimes I tend to get so depressed I just lay in the bed or am out of it. She [her psychiatrist] told me to try to do something that I like, that I enjoy." When Cindy is asked if she talks with her psychiatrist about her issues (she was sexually molested by her stepfather and has since been diagnosed with BPD with psychotic features), she says, "Yes," but then quickly reveals that the content of their discussions is similarly limited to "how I am feeling today. She asks if I am doing any better. How my day is going. How do I feel? Do I feel up or down?" When Joelle is asked whether her psychiatrist has ever asked about her history of sexual abuse, she replied, "No," and described how the focus of sessions with her psychiatrist was on "what's happening now" and "getting me the medication." Rachel's sole mental health care provider is a psychiatrist with a similarly limited role in treating Rachel's schizophrenia. As a result, Rachel says that when she gets "out of balance," she has developed her own strategies for dealing with hallucinations and delusions, including self-taught versions of mindful awareness techniques.

We did find, however, a handful of exceptions, that is, women who are also receiving some therapeutic counseling from their psychiatrists. Marisol, who has been diagnosed with OCD, sees a psychiatrist who not only manages her drug treatment but also provides some very basic cognitive behavioral therapy in the form of offering coping strategies that Marisol can use. Marisol illustrates these techniques: "If you count like five times, count three times. Say, 'I don't have to do it. Everything is fine. My mind's trying to play with me. Just don't do it.'"

A handful of the women interviewed for this study were using counseling services only. Charlene, who has been in recovery for drug and alcohol addiction and is currently battling severe depression and anxiety, is one of those participants who are not receiving psychiatric services. In Charlene's case, this choice is specific, based on her legitimate concerns over chemical dependence, and one that is supported by her addiction counselor and psychologist. When asked how she views her overall experiences with therapy, Charlene replies, "It's positive." In groups, she says, "You receive a lot and I contribute a lot . . . [and] it's pretty good." When asked about the forms of therapy that she has been receiving, the response is "cognitive behavioral, coping skills, and coping situations." What these have taught her is to "take a deep breath and analyze the situation," a technique she finds useful in managing her anxiety.

Improvements

In relation to psychiatric drug usage, a significant question is whether women who were prescribed such drugs felt they have experienced mood, cognitive, or other improvements as a result of usage. Although the majority felt they had either received no benefit or experienced an adverse side effect, several women stated they felt mentally, emotionally, or physically better than they had prior to embarking on a psychiatric drug regimen. Deborah is one: "I'm on depression meds . . . [whispers] and I feel so much better." Valerie and Cindy have similarly been diagnosed with major depression and feel better when taking their antidepressants. When asked, the latter simply says, "The meds are helpful."

Looking at the statements made by women who noted positive reactions to prescribed treatments, we discovered that "feeling better" is largely synonymous with symptom abatement, a phenomenon that is not easy to dismiss, given the suffering that such symptoms often entail for the individual. As the historian Andrew Scull has remarked, "if, for some of those who suffer from the miseries madness brings in its train, antipsychotics, antidepressants, and anti-anxiety drugs provide . . . advantages, we should not dismiss them out of hand" (2011, p. 121). Certainly, the women who have found an easing or cessation of their symptoms would disagree with any attempt at characterizing the benefits they feel they derive from psychiatric drugs as placebo effects. Marybeth is a case in point. Having been diagnosed with BPD, she was placed on the drug lamotrigine. Although she is still experiencing periods where she "gets a little anxious," after six months of taking the drug, her mood is elevated and she is "not suicidal anymore." Such results undoubtedly represent a positive development for someone who has made an estimated eight to sixteen suicide attempts. Eden, a recovering alcoholic, believes that her continuing sobriety is due to "the anxiety meds, [because] I definitely need those." Now that she is calmer under the influence of the anxiolytic drugs she is taking, she no longer feels the need to self-medicate with alcohol. Again, the drug's effect is no small thing in the life of someone who has struggled with alcohol addiction.

What is of some interest is that some women are somewhat cognizant of the fact that the drugs they are taking are producing sedating effects that put a damper on their thoughts and behaviors. Not only do several of the women recognize these effects, but such effects are seen as beneficial. As an example, Marybeth notes that lamotrigine places her in a state where she is now "learning to tolerate things." The word she uses to describe this state is *numb*. She acknowledges the fact that she feels "so numb" and that it is "not real . . . [and] not natural." Amber, who is also on lamotrigine, similarly notes that the drug slows down her thought processes, an effect that became particularly notable when the recommended dosage was doubled: "It helps a lot," she states. "I don't think about things like I used to." Instead, she can now "let things go." Although Marvella is no longer experiencing delusional thoughts following her move to Los Angeles, her insomnia is exacerbated by her present living conditions. Sharing close quarters with strangers has been making her particularly irritable and she has become "very quick to temper." Although Marvella recognizes that the antidepressant she is taking, sertraline, is not a panacea, she feels she is now better able to manage her temper and to accept people for who they are. "Why worry or stress out about something you can't do anything about?" she asks, adding, "I think the pills, they help me to a degree." When Meredith is asked how she deals with the feelings of anger, anxiousness, or depression she experiences while living in the shelter, she replies, "I take my medication." Felicia is frank about her use of quetiapine and the benefits she derives from it: "I used to take a pretty large amount, [so] that I would be passed out for more than a day [laughing]. I was kind of enjoying it so much, my doctor would ask me and I wouldn't say anything."

The responses of Meredith and these other women call to mind Vincent Lyon-Callo's comments concerning the biopsychiatrization of homelessness:

> Homeless people (like many other people in the US) are being medicated as a method of treating their "mental illness." Any contributions that social inequality and related systemic conditions play in the process of depression, for example, are transformed into bio-chemical disorders of the mind and of the individualized self. Why feel anguish or depression when one can be sedated with one of the many new psychotropic medications? Why examine systemic contributions to depression when one can simply homogenize brain functioning and, through the process of sedation, marginalize discontent as a mental illness? (2008, p. 62)

Kathy, like Meredith and several others, is clear about the fact that much of her current unhappiness is based on unresolved issues from her past, coupled with the miserable situation in which she finds herself as an impoverished woman. She too acknowledges that the major benefit she derives from psychiatric drugs is not the righting of a chemical imbalance but rather the real or perceived ability to blunt some of the mental and emotional pain she routinely experiences. Referring to the misery of living in her shelter, she says, "There's so many people in here, it's stressful. It's depressing . . . [and] I don't like waking up and knowing I need to take a Zoloft because I'm going to be really upset about something. Something is going to happen."

Although symptom abatement is frequently cited as a primary reason why some women view psychiatric drugs as helpful, clearly, for a smaller number, these drugs are seen as serving a deeper, more profound purpose. In the stories of this latter group, antidepressants, antipsychotics, and other drugs are components of programs of self-improvement, tools to aid individuals in either returning to their former states or as a means of facilitating opportunities to realize what is believed to be their true selves (Rose 2007). Erica is among those who express such sentiments. When she entered psychiatric treatment, Erica was placed on five different drugs for OCD, depression, and anxiety. She worked with a psychiatrist on finding what was felt to be an appropriate drug combination and dosage levels and today credits her current drug regimen for increasing her ability to be independent. Prior to entering the domain of biopsychiatry, Erica says of herself, "I couldn't take a shower by myself, eat by myself." Today, "I'm getting better." To illustrate, she notes how she has been able to turn her life around: "Now I work. I eat. I take a shower by myself." Deborah is also among those wanting a life transformation. As a child she was raised in a physically abusive home in which she both watched her mother being beaten and was beaten herself. Years spent wrestling with an addiction to crack cocaine led to unsuccessful stints in recovery programs and an ongoing struggle to stop using before Deborah turned to a local mental health clinic for help. There she was prescribed antidepressants. Now in her early fifties and sober for some months, she is in individual, group, and family therapeutic programs and feels that her life has substantially turned around. She credits the antidepressants with elevating her mood to the point where she can stay in counseling and maintain sobriety: "Now that I have my mood elevator, I feel more focused." She is working on a plan to get her cosmetology license and wants to start a charity program to help battered and homeless women regain their self-esteem. The extent to which Deborah attributes the positive changes in her life to the effects of fluoxetine is evident in how she speaks about the need for women to educate themselves about mental health issues:

> I think a lot of women need to understand, especially in this high-stress society we live in, we have to understand that we have some degree of mental illness. How could you not? It's better to understand it, and, if necessary, get medication . . . be open to it. It's not a shame factor. I'd rather say I'm on depression meds than be on the street smoking crack.

Deborah's story also illustrates another point: women in this group often believed that the act of taking a pill is not sufficient for achieving personal reform; they must also exert effort to achieve transformation (see Rose 2007). Ella exemplifies this belief. Diagnosed with schizoaffective disorder and on antipsychotic drugs, Ella says of them, "It's working because I want it to work. I don't want to lay around like a vegetable and just . . . [be] helpless . . . [and] I want it to work." For Kathy personal reform is a learning process, and what she has learned is that "your meds can only do so much." Thus, if she wishes to stay "on an even plane," she must "combine the help" of her psychiatrist and her psychologist and make use of every available opportunity for self-improvement.

Worth noting is that some of those women who felt they were receiving positive benefits from their use of prescription drugs, particularly in the case of antidepressants, were quite possibly experiencing a placebo effect. The possibility that the efficacy of antidepressants might be attributable to the power of suggestion is well known and often discussed within the psy sciences literature (Gueorguieva, Mallinckrodt, and Krystal 2011; Kirsch 2010; Walsh et al. 2002). However, few, if any researchers, have remarked on what this placebo effect might look like for individual women, particularly those within impoverished communities who experience high rates of depression and are therefore among those most likely to be prescribed antidepressants. The prescribing standard is to instruct patients to take their recommended dose on a daily basis in order for it to be effective, unless the individual is being tapered off the drug, but we found that in discussing their drug usage, several of the women who ascribed positive effects to the antidepressants they were taking revealed they had not actually been taking them consistently, as recommended. Cora, a fifty-eight-year-old woman who is battling depression over both illness and her experience of being homeless for the first time, is a case in point. She has been prescribed sertraline, which, she says, "mellows me out when I really feel depressed about how I feel." In discussing her use, Cora reveals that she doesn't follow the doctor's orders because "I find that if I take it too much and it gets into my system I feel paranoid. I start thinking delusional. So I have to take it in moderation . . . unless I'm totally depressed and down, and I absolutely have to, then I take it." How often is this? "Maybe twice a week." Stella, a sixty-year-old woman diagnosed with PTSD and depression, had also been prescribed sertraline. Her story, another tale of beneficial effects, is also strongly suggestive of the power of placebo: "I had a bad incident one time. I told my psychiatrist that I doubled the Zoloft. I took one in the morning and one at night. She said take it in the morning. So for a whole week I did that. They monitored me, and after one week we stopped. I'm back to normal." Sandra is another woman who has been diagnosed with PTSD and placed on an antidepressant. She doesn't recall the name of the pill, only that "it's an oval [and] I'm supposed to take it one in the morning, one in the afternoon." Like Cora, Sandra only takes a pill "if I know it's gonna be a bad one and my day has gone bad and I'm having these episodes. I take it before I flip out or go have a nervous breakdown." Her success with the drug is intermittent: sometimes it works and she feels better, and other times "it's a couple of hours later and I'm still with my back up."

Nothing, Not Much, or Worse

Although some women found benefits in using psychiatric drugs, a significant number reported either no improvement or even negative side effects. In relation to the former, when Tess is asked if the antidepressants she was prescribed were helpful in dealing with her low moods, she replies, "No, they were not helpful at all." As a result, Tess stopped taking the pills. Jan, who had taken herself off of fluoxetine, felt that the only effect she received from the drug was that it made her lose weight. In terms of elevating her feelings of depression following her mother's death, she noted that she felt no better. "It's the same if you take an aspirin a day, or whatever they say it is, but that aspirin really isn't doing nothing." When Chris confided that she had begun seeing what she termed a "therapist" four months previously, she was asked about the nature of the therapy sessions:

> LAURA: What would the therapist do? Just listen?
> CHRIS: No, give me some more medicine.
> LAURA: Does the medication help you?
> CHRIS: No.

Some of the women reported side effects that included a worsening of existing symptoms or the development of new health problems. Rachel said that as a consequence of taking quetiapine, she has become psychologically dependent on it: "When I don't have any, then I tell myself, 'I can't sleep!' Then right there and then, I can't sleep!" When Jan told her psychiatrist that fluoxetine was having no effect on her beyond weight loss, she was prescribed a higher dosage: "She said maybe 'cause it's suppressing your appetite. We'll up the dosage.' And I thought, 'Up the dosage?' So I went with it, and it was like I was taking methamphetamine." When asked to clarify how the increased dosage made her feel, Jan makes the sound of a car's engine revving, adding, "My mind was racing, so I don't want any more of that." Joanne, who was diagnosed with PTSD, was prescribed "an anxiety pill for stress." Although she does not recall which drug she was prescribed, she complained about the fact that she was experiencing negative side effects, including a fifteen- to twenty-pound weight gain in three months: "The doctor said, 'Oh, no, that doesn't happen.'" Tess had a similar reaction to quetiapine, which she was given inside prison: her weight rapidly increased and she became borderline diabetic. Of the drug, she says that it increased her appetite and she was "eating sugar."

One of the purported benefits of the newer range of antipsychotic drugs is that they are said to lead to fewer serious debilitating side effects than the first-generation drugs, such as chlorpromazine (Gardos 1999). That said, they too come with their own potentially adverse effects, including the movement disorders (such as limb stiffness, mask-like faces, restlessness, and agitation) noted with the previous generation of drugs (Correll and Schenk 2008). Thus, whereas weight gain and other negative metabolic effects were more commonly cited by the women in this study, a small minority said they were having issues such as repetitive muscle spasms or were even observed to be twitching or constantly moving during the interview. Paula exemplifies the former: diagnosed with PTSD and BPDs, she was previously placed on quetiapine but was subsequently removed from it and put on doxepin instead when she developed motor dysfunction. As she explains of quetiapine, "you get them twitches in your knee when you take it!" Although Alex never addresses the issue of whether she is experiencing any adverse side effects from the psychiatric drugs she is taking, risperidone and lamotrigine, Alex is ceaselessly in motion, even while seated and presumably relaxed.

The primary effect of many psychiatric drugs is sedation. In some cases sedation is perceived to be a desirable consequence of taking a given drug in that it prevents women from feeling depressed or anxious about their current situation or about past experiences. For others, though, sedation is a significant negative effect that they neither wanted nor sought. Prior to entering a shelter, Lois was living with her father and attending therapeutic services on an outpatient basis for PTSD that she developed in response to the physical and sexual assaults she had experienced. During this time she was in group therapy and had been placed on psychiatric drugs. Of the two, she says that "the counselling worked better than the meds." She was so effectively sedated by the latter that "when my brother came to visit . . . I don't even remember him coming, and it broke my heart."

Not surprisingly, women who either experienced no beneficial effects from the psychiatric drugs they had been prescribed or were left to deal with negative side effects frequently reported they had stopped taking their pills.

They became, in psychiatric parlance, "treatment noncompliant." Such was the case with Joanne, who experienced not only adverse metabolic effects from a drug she described as an "anxiety pill for stress" but also changes in mood that made her so miserable she stopped taking it. Subsequently, Joanne's girlfriend told her, "'You seemed more like a monster when you were on that pill. Instead of it helping you, it was making it worse.'" The pool of noncompliant individuals was not, however, limited to individuals like Joanne. It also included women who had been prescribed a drug and refused to take it or women who would not even countenance receiving a prescription. None of what we found is unusual: studies suggest that as many as one-third to one-half of patients are noncompliant with psychiatric drug treatment.

Aside from their own experiences of null or negative effects, women typically reported at least one of several other reasons why they opted to become noncompliant. First were concerns that arose from observing the effects of psychoactive drugs on others. Given the extent to which homeless citizens are treated with such drugs, the majority of women living in shelters or on the streets encounter a relatively large number of individuals on psychiatric drug regimens. As a consequence, they are exposed to multiple close-range opportunities to see the possible deleterious effects of these drugs on others, and so many do not want to experience those effects firsthand. For example, Diane acknowledges, "I've got mental issues," but feels she can handle them without having to "soak myself in drugs." Referring to some of the people in her shelter who were on psychiatric drugs, she says, "I see a lot of people around here walking like a zombie. I'm like, 'What are they on? I don't want it.'" Jan, who has removed herself from fluoxetine and refuses to take other psychoactive drugs, is concerned about their effects. "Lots of that medicine got bad side effects to it." She adds, "Most people I know that take Seroquel, Prozac, their kidneys and livers are failing, and I'm not going to go through that. I don't need that."

A recurring theme in the literature on treatment noncompliance is the idea of dependency: that is, the fear among psychiatric patients that they could become physically, mentally, or emotionally dependent on psychiatric drugs. This fear was voiced by several of the women who had stopped taking prescribed drugs or refused to take them as prescribed. Margaret was on her way to a job interview when she met Laura in the church of a local shelter. Dressed in business attire, she looked anything but how she felt: "I'm clinically depressed right now." When asked if she had been taking antidepressants, her response is quick: "No, I choose not to. I don't want to get dependent on any meds." As is noted earlier in this chapter, Margaret's fears of dependency are not wholly unwarranted. Women, including women with preexisting histories of addiction, are sometimes prescribed dependency-producing drugs by physicians (Huey, Fthenos, and Hryniewicz 2012).

Some women refused to take the psychiatric drugs prescribed for them on the grounds that they were either misdiagnosed or prescribed a type of drug that would not be helpful to them. As may be recalled, Candice, who had sought help for obsessional thinking and an inability to focus, disputes the diagnosis of major depression she was given. To treat her depression, Candice was prescribed the drug aripiprazole, which is often used as an adjunctive treatment in treating major depression. She says, "You sit there. You are explaining, and you understand what you are saying to them, and they just tell you, 'Well, I'm going to prescribe you Abilify.' Abilify is an amplifier for another antidepressant, and they just give it to me just because. They say, 'Just give it a try,' and I just clearly said, 'I'm not a depressed person.'" Candice opted not to take the drug. As a result of these and other experiences, she is now firmly of the view that "going to these mental health places is a joke."

Somewhat ironically, given that psychiatric drugs are frequently touted as a foundational block in the effort to help homeless citizens improve their lives, several women spoke of how the use of these drugs is actually counterproductive to self-improvement and other desired goals. In talking about her future, Yvonne radiates excitement over the fact that she has recently started school and begun an exercise class. She has been prescribed psychoactive drugs to treat depression and anxiety but refuses to take them because she does not want to do anything that might affect her ability to function in school or in her other activities: "I don't want to be walking around like a zombie." In speaking of the effects of psychiatric drugs on others, Kit says, "I see it all the time, period . . . [that] certain medicines you take affect your mind, especially if your mental capacity can't handle it . . . [and] it have [other women] like muted." Psychiatric drugs, she believes, "mess with your mind, so that you can't speak or talk." Rather than seeing them as therapeutically beneficial, Kit is of the view that these drugs are prescribed because "[the doctors] don't understand what's the matter . . . [and] they don't know how to handle situations like that." So their response, she says, is to "put you on medicine to try to get rid of it." This strategy fails to work "because they haven't got to the root of the problem." Kit believes that too often psychiatrists "don't want to take time to get to the root of the problem," so they give patients "something to cover it up." Kit is a firm believer that what "people need is someone they can trust and that they can talk to." For Kit, as for others, psychoactive drugs are not a solution to help move one forward but an additional barrier. Jan agrees. Describing herself on quetiapine, she says it made her "zombie out all day . . . so I quit taking it."

Despite the fact many of the women interviewed for this project had been on psychiatric drugs for years and had been either physically or sexually assaulted while on the streets, only Mercy, near the end of the project, raises what should have been an obvious issue, as a criminologist, to consider from the beginning: the highly sedating effects of these drugs, particularly when taken during the day, can render women vulnerable to victimization. Mercy raises this concern when discussing why she refuses to take her prescription for quetiapine, except for the four days prior to a psychiatric visit: "They gave me this one thing that knocked me out. I went, 'I can't take this drug during the daytime. I want to be aware.'" Coincidentally, the interview with Mercy came right after a hurried conversation with another female member of the research team, who was feeling awkward after noticing that several of the men at this shelter were openly staring at her crotch. With this conversation in mind, Laura clarified with Mercy if, when she said she wanted "to be aware" of her surroundings, she was concerned for her physical safety. Nodding vigorously, Mercy is quick to reply, "And the guys here they watch . . . they watch." Elise, who had been sexually assaulted while living on the streets, observes that "a woman on the streets is marked for any predator . . . [and] it's a constant watch." Elise had made the conscious choice to take the drugs prescribed for her, citalopram, quetiapine, and clozapine, at night before bed because she felt safer being sedated in the shelter than she did on the street. Referring to the morning "med call," she notes, "I don't want to take something here and [then] be knocked out." For Elise, the streets are a terrible place for a woman on psychiatric drugs because she has to be alert all the time in order to avoid being victimized. Zoe is equally terrified of the men and the women who reside in her shelter, fearing that several are violent and may victimize her. She was originally on aripiprazole but was switched to lamotrigine because of her safety concerns: "I don't want to be a zombie around here."

In many instances, women were advised by their psychiatrist or primary care physician to only take highly sedating drugs in the evening, prior to going to bed. For the women in secure shelters, this practice would, in theory, remove some of the opportunity for threat. However, this is not universally the case: some women had histories of sleeping rough,[6] and others were advised to take sedating drugs during the day. Nicole, who is on a regimen of levetiracetam, olanzapine, and lithium, had until very recently been sleeping under trees and the freeway system with a friend while taking at least two drugs with sedative effects. The threat of constant victimization she had been facing in this precarious situation is indirectly referenced when discussing how happy she is to be in the shelter and away from the men in the streets who, she notes, "like to intimidate." Although Nicole does not specify how or when the violence occurred, she does acknowledge that she has been both physically and sexually assaulted as an adult, neither event occurring within the context of a domestic violence situation. Lindsay has been secure at night in a shelter; however, she is one of the women advised to take sedating drugs during the day, when women are generally asked to leave most shelters. Lindsay is not only taking five milligrams of clonazepam daily but is also taking the maximum daily dose of quetiapine (600 milligrams in the evening and another 200 milligrams in the morning). Not surprisingly, she complains of finding alertness early in the day difficult: "In the morning, I'm so worn out." Sharisse is staying in the same mixed-gender facility that some of the other women have variously described as "hell," "scary," and "not safe." Diagnosed with major depression and dealing with panic attacks, for the past year Sharisse has been taking three drugs: aripiprazole (five milligrams), trazodone (100 milligrams at night), and risperidone (50 milligrams twice daily). Although the effects of these drugs at these doses will vary depending on the individual, worth noting is that the risperidone alone, which Sharisse takes morning and evening, can have highly sedative effects and lower psychomotor functioning.[7] On the streets, impairment in a vulnerable female represents a significant safety risk. For example, when we arrive at the shelter at which Kerry is staying, the med call is already under way. As we walk up to the front gate, someone calls out, "Hey, Miss Laura." Standing by the gate is Kerry among a small group of men. As we greet her, it's obvious that the woman who was so funny and "with it" during her interview is now acting like a zombie, mumbling her words, and unable to focus. A research team member, who had also made Kerry's acquaintance the previous visit, later confirms that Kerry, who is diligent about taking her prescription for aripiprazole, had been counteracting its sedating effects by smoking crack. When we had last seen her, she had been flush with money and had been routinely smoking, thus a very different demeanor. On this day, Kerry's money must have run out. Two hours later, as we are leaving the shelter, she is still standing by the front gate. When we try to say good-bye to her, she no longer seems to recognize Laura.

Does Anyone Get Better?

In reviewing the interview transcripts, we found that some women do report positive effects, including improvements in mood and reductions in hallucinations or delusory beliefs. To what extent such improvements are the result of placebo effects, we cannot say; thus, we acknowledge that some people do achieve symptom abatement, and symptom abatement alone causes them to feel marginally, somewhat, or significantly better. In many other cases, however, the same drugs have a null or detrimental effect on an individual's well-being, leading a number of individuals to stop taking them.

Thus far, we have been looking at two of the groups discussed above. But a third group has much to tell us about how psychiatric drugs may or may not work in treating the problems of homeless citizens. In this group are women like Deborah and Kathy, who choose to take psychiatric drugs as part of a program of personal reformation and who report significant positive benefits from doing so. Their stories are instructive here because of the reform-oriented work they were undertaking: these women were engaged in multiple forms of therapeutic treatment simultaneously. Deborah, who says she feels "so much better" from taking antidepressants, also receives individual counseling on a weekly basis, participates in family therapy, and is active in both her church and the community. In talking about engaging in church and volunteer activities, her face lights up, and she shares her dream of getting a cosmetology license and starting a volunteer "beauty program" for homeless women. Kathy, the woman who takes mood stabilizing drugs to "slow down" her brain and talks a mile a minute while her brain "spiders" from topic to topic, reports that the drugs are helping her to feel on a more "even plane" and that she is feeling better and more positive as a result. Like Deborah, the extent to which psychiatric drugs alone are responsible for Kathy's increased well-being is debatable. Kathy and her husband, who is also at the shelter, are enrolled in a variety of individual and group therapy programs, some of which are specifically trauma informed and also include art and relationship workshops. These groups give her a new and more positive focus, and she happily states, "I can go to groups all day, every day." Such examples suggest drugs do not play the central role in fostering individual improvements, but rather drugs in combination with therapy, especially in conjunction with positive changes in interpersonal relationships and in one's social environment, bring about the greatest change.

Vanessa, who has recently started seeing a psychiatrist, expresses similar thoughts. In describing the current state of her treatment sessions, she says they are oriented toward "Let's find the right medication for you." Although she appreciates the relief that the drugs provide from the thoughts and feelings that often overwhelm her, she offers the following thought: "I really don't think medication is the answer completely. I think it's helped as far as for sleeping and to keep my crying at bay, and you know, my anxiety, it's gone down a little bit, but I don't think it's the answer." What is the answer? "I think with enough counseling and enough, you know, coaching, and [being] given coping skills to deal with the stuff that's happened in the past, I can move forward." She adds, "But as long as that doesn't happen, I'm not getting anywhere." Jan agrees. Of the drugs, she says, "It makes it worse, and any trauma you're dealing with, it suppresses it. You don't want to suppress it. You want to talk it out, so you can overcome it, not stay there. And the way that they treat you, you stay where you at. You don't overcome; you just add to it." Like several others, Donna does not see drugs as the solution to what she sees as emotional problems: "I don't have to take pills to calm me down. I need someone to talk to. I need therapy. That's what I need. I don't want pills." Having completed detox and rehab for a decades-long drug addiction, she scorned the idea of a drug-based solution: "It's like, you go into detox and what do they give me? Pills." Grace, who is a firm believer in biopsychiatry and speaks knowledgeably of her "chemical imbalance," remains, however, somewhat skeptical of much of the treatment she had received from the medical community. She had spent years searching for help from both primary care physicians and psychiatrists for her low moods and suicidal feelings. Of her visits to one particular general practitioner, she says, "He gives you Xanax. They just write the prescription and you're out." Then this smiling woman adds in a noticeably darker tone, "It takes you fifty years to get the appointment, and then when you get the appointment, all they do is write the prescription . . . [so] they get paid for writing prescriptions and no one ever gets well."

The Power to Prescribe

When physicians prescribe a course of treatment for a patient, parameters of professional conduct allow for the assumption that they typically do so under the conviction that the proposed treatment will either heal the patients' conditions or otherwise ease or end patients' suffering. Of course, we must recognize our study is limited in that we do not include the perspective of the prescribers (we did not interview the persons who treated the homeless women in our study), and thus we cannot speak to their views, experiences, positioning, and frustrations in their professional activities nor their views toward their treatment of female clients who are homeless. Nonetheless, although the two things are frequently conflated, healing and prescription are not synonymous. In the case of biopsychiatric treatment, this fact is well understood; that psychoactive drugs do not cure patients is generally recognized (National Institute of Mental Health 2014). Instead, their use is limited to reducing or suppressing the positive symptoms associated with specific conditions. Suppression of symptoms is not healing in any conventional sense of the word. Thus, although the power to heal and the act of prescribing are not one and the same, the authority to prescribe treatment, sanctioned as it is by the state and organized as part of an expert knowledge discourse, is still a significant form of power and one that remains exclusive to physicians and a small range of other healthcare professionals.

The power to prescribe manifests in various forms through the therapeutic encounter. It is manifest, for example, when patients specifically consult psychiatrists to receive a remedy for their problems, on the basis of the latter's expert knowledge of mental health conditions and treatments. It is also manifest in the faith that patients place in the prescriptive advice they receive from their doctors and their willingness to follow that advice, even when they dispute its utility.

The willingness to accept biopsychiatric prescription is fostered not only by the faith we generally place in experts and in medical science but also by the very nature of the contact between patient and doctor. In mental health settings, patients typically encounter psychiatrists or primary care physicians because they are in a state of distress, suffering from emotional, cognitive, and behavioral difficulties that may be overwhelming. In this regard, the patient is uniquely vulnerable to the power to prescribe. In relation to the willingness of patients to follow advice regarding psychiatric drug treatment they might not otherwise wish to take, Duncan Double notes: "Medication is often prescribed in life crises and serves to reinforce defensive mechanisms against overwhelming anxiety. When people are desperate they will accept almost anything that is proposed to help them" (2011, p. 200).

In describing the patient-psychiatrist relationship, one notable critic of present psychiatric practices has observed that "your psychiatrist will have more power than you" (Breggin 1991, p. 16). If this observation is true of the general population, then one must accept that homeless women are uniquely vulnerable in this regard. Certainly, they live in highly adverse situations under stressful conditions. Thus, these women who, lacking the opportunity or wherewithal to remove themselves from those conditions, are desperate for solutions to the problems they face. Evidence of such desperation can be found in the stories of Meredith and Teneka, among others, who use the sedative effects of the prescribed drugs as relief from the stresses of shelter life. Further, as noted in the preceding chapter, the ranks of homeless citizens are filled with underprivileged women, who lack equal social standing and equal access to expert knowledge, and who exist within institutions and a larger society that privilege the type of knowledge and power wielded by medical professionals. As a result of these power disparities, when a medical professional tells a woman that her problems are caused by an imbalance in neurochemical transmitters, she may be more willing to uncritically accept this truth and any proposed remedy, including the seemingly easy fix of psychoactive drugs, particularly if other solutions have failed. Such is the case with Grace, who had spent years battling depression and addiction without success and whose latest diagnosis and prescriptions came as the result of a second confinement in a psychiatric institution. Lastly, and as we detail more fully in the next chapter, homeless women cycle through various institutions that not only endorse biopsychiatry's prescriptive power but actively take steps to obtain client compliance, and we describe the aftereffects of structural violence, stigma, and society's dedication to the allopathic medical model—cuts and chemicals—in this regard.

Notes

1. In psychiatric parlance, *positive* is used to describe symptoms that are present among those typically diagnosed with a delusion disorder and that are viewed as excessive or distorted when compared to so-called normal functioning (i.e., delusions and hallucinations). By way of contrast, "negative" symptoms are those that signify a lessening of normal functions (i.e., flat affect and alogia [poverty of speech]).

2. Lamotrigine is primarily used for treating seizures but has been used as a mood stabilizer.

3. Chlorpromazine is a phenothiazine antipsychotic medicine that can be taken orally or injected.

4. Riperidone, a benzisoxazole derivative classified as an atypical antipsychotic, has a long history of use for treating schizophrenia.

5. Lorazepam, part of the benzodiazepine group, is used to treat anxiety.

6. As may be recalled from the last chapter, one reason women might sleep rough is as a result of losing their place in shelters due to policies regarding maximum length of stay.

7. This point about the highly sedating effects of Risperdal (risperidone) was demonstrated in a study in which twelve healthy, adult male volunteers were dosed with two milligrams of Risperdal and 50 milligrams of chlorpromazine, respectively (Hughes, Lynch, and Yates 1999). Seven of the twelve study participants reported greater lethargy with the Risperdal and exhibited a greater level of impairment in psychomotor performance (Hughes, Lynch, and Yates 1999).

6

The Issue of Compliance

A small line has formed at the entrance to the large dining hall. Women are standing there, watching us, waiting for one of the research team to signal that we are ready for the next interviewee. The next person in line is Hannah, a thirty-five-year-old African American woman. As we walk to the interview space, her nose is running, she moves slowly, and she appears to have toilet paper wadded up in each of her ears. Without immediately asking about the toilet paper, the interviewer, Laura, makes a point to raise her voice slightly and speak in clear tones. Hannah answers each question, which indicates she can hear. However, the responses come slowly and in incomplete sentences; she is demonstrating alogia, a speech pattern marked by missing words and incomplete thoughts, commonly associated with the diagnosis of schizophrenia. For example, when asked about the effects of the medications she is taking, she responds, "More manageable. I learned that I take them every single day . . . and . . . unh . . . in the event that I feel that something more is going on, they want to add more medication . . . it kind of speeds up the . . . unh . . . the . . . recovery, the healing process better. Continue. Stay on your meds." None of the antipsychotic drugs treat alogia, including the two she is taking: perphenazine and risperidone. The other effects of these drugs are evident in the slow rate at which she moves. However, the toilet paper remains puzzling. Finally, I point out, "I noticed that you have some hearing aids or something in your ears." To which Hannah replies, "I'm just getting over a minor cold." Instead of expressing confusion, I simply nod my head.[1]

One way to make sense of Hannah's odd statement would be to suppose that she had not been taking the drugs as prescribed, but that is not the case. Hannah has been faithfully taking her pills for several years, following participation in a community-based "mental health recovery program." Within such programs, compliance with prescribed drug treatments is actively encouraged through a variety of techniques used by program workers. One such technique is to pair the receipt of disability benefits or income funds with taking drugs dispensed by a community health worker (a program informally termed a "med and money drop") (Brodwin 2010). In Hannah's case, she was enrolled in a program for four years that drew on further strategies to foster client compliance: educational seminars and group activities aimed at spreading the message of so-called patient responsibility. This message is reinforced through participation in peer support groups, as the following exchange with Hannah illustrates:

> HANNAH: They would teach us coping skills and triggers and make sure we were taking our meds.
> Laura: You found that useful?
> Hannah: Yeah.
> Laura: Do you use any of those tools they gave you?
> Hannah: I use my support system. Taking my meds. Just . . . staying responsible . . . things like that.

Because Hannah has been effectively responsibilized into diligently taking her prescribed drugs, she has not been subject to any of the more coercive measures that can be employed to enforce compliance. Others have been less fortunate.

Although we clearly acknowledge again that what society thinks of as helping institutions, such as shelters, do provide necessary and fundamental supports for the women they serve by providing care and sustenance and allowing women a roof over their heads rather than forcing them to sleep rough, including at times without strings attached (see Cloke, May, and Johnsen 2010; DeVerteuil and Wilton 2009; Gowan 2010), we here speak to the abeyance, control, and surveillance—the coercive care (see Johnsen and Fitzapatrick 2010)—that is too often part and parcel of shelter living. In the pages that follow, we explore the range of persuasive and coercive techniques used to garner individual compliance with psychiatric drug regimens. As documented below, these techniques are utilized within and across a number of institutions. Indeed, we find strategies of compliance within the policies and practices of shelters, hospitals, prisons, probation offices, community mental health centers, and state mental health facilities, and these strategies are variously supported through court orders or the ministrations of community nurses and shelter workers, each of whom work individually and in concert to try to garner both individuals' acquiescence to and their active participation in drug treatment plans.[2]

Shelters

Shelters play an important role in the psychiatrization of homelessness (Lyon-Callo 2008). To illustrate, we look at the work of the case manager, who has the responsibility of helping women identify individual needs and facilitating access to appropriate services. In this capacity, shelter case managers often single out mental health issues as a potential barrier to securing employment and housing and therefore routinely recommend clients receive diagnosis and treatment (see also Lyon-Callo 2008). Indeed, evidence of this process at work can be found in several of the stories already presented. One of these was Nikki's account (in Chapter 1), in which she reported having been lay-diagnosed with major depression by a shelter case manager. This particular case manager did not simply refer her to the shelter's doctor for treatment but also recommended a specific treatment modality: a prescription of sertraline. Jan had a similar experience with a case manager at a different shelter. When asked if she had experienced any pressure to take psychiatric drugs, Jan acknowledged receiving pressure from her shelter case manager: "They wanted me to go to Downtown Mental Health, and I said, 'No, I don't wanna take medication. Medication ain't gonna do nothing.'" Over the past seven years of her homelessness, the Pastor has also been referred to several mental health centers by the various shelters she has used in order to seek biopsychiatric treatment. When asked about the role of the shelter staff in this process, the Pastor is direct: "They've pushed it on me. In the shelters, they had me taking all kinds of medicine." Referring to the shelter at which she is presently residing, she says, "They're pushers. And then you can't get help. That's how I ended up in a place down on Broadway. They told me I have to go to a psychiatrist. He gives me drugs and then when I refused to take it, [they say,] 'We can't help you.'"

Within shelters, psychiatric drug treatment not only is viewed as a tool for helping women overcome mental health issues but is also seen by some case managers as useful for quelling problem behaviors within the facility. Donna represents the type of individual for whom sedation might seem an attractive option. Having spent years living on the streets and in crack houses, she is a highly confrontational, combative individual with a history of getting into fights with roommates at her shelter, a fact she openly acknowledges. Indeed, not only was she aggressive toward the researcher during the interview, but one of her former roommates advised that Donna had to be moved to another room when she began issuing threats following a theft incident. Donna was also impervious to the threat of being thrown out of the shelter for violence: "I don't let no bitch in here disrespect me. I'm not going to stand there and argue with them. I'm going to slap them around." As a result of continuing interpersonal problems between Donna and other residents, her case manager called her into his office for a discussion.[3] Describing the meeting, she says, "My case manager told me I had to see mental health." When asked why, her answer reflects institutional concerns: "Because he says I'm bumping heads." When subsequently asked, "Is he telling you, you need pills?" she replies, "Yeah."

Shelters also facilitate treatment compliance through on-site arrangements they establish with local mental health centers. For example, a shelter in the valley has psychiatric staff from one such center visit residents of their facility twice a week. The purpose of these visits is revealed when Stella is asked about whether she is receiving therapeutic counseling along with her prescriptions of risperidone, trazodone, and sertraline. "No," she answers, but she wishes that she was because "sometimes you just want to let it all out." Instead, the psychiatrists who visit have been focused on monitoring her dosages. When asked if she sees them as helpful in terms of addressing her issues, Stella dodges the question, replying, "Both of them are very, very nice to me." Like several other women at this shelter, Stella is on so many psychiatric and other drugs (for various health conditions) that when the subject of her use of psychiatric services first arose during the interview, she too was carrying a list of all of the drugs currently prescribed to her.

Ostensibly set up to ensure that residents do not lose their prescription drugs or have them stolen, some shelters have also created med calls, designated times during which workers dispense and oversee the consumption of residents' drugs. Med calls are typically held in the morning and evening. The process at one shelter was described to me as follows:

> SARA: They have a medicine cabinet. . . . You get your meds, take your meds, that's it.
>
> LAURA: Do they watch the dosage?
>
> SARA: They do because they don't want people getting other people's meds, so they watch you from the moment you go in the cabinet to get your meds, put 'em on the table, take 'em out right in front of them, sign off, take them back.

Although depicted by Sara as a benign, even helpful process, the reality is that this transaction is documented, therefore empowering shelter staff to conduct surveillance on whether individual residents are complying with treatment. This monitoring can have negative consequences for women who are not treatment compliant.[4]

Social Security

Given their impoverished situations, most of the women in this study were on some form of income support or in the process of seeking income assistance through one or more state programs. Of these, the most commonly referenced were federal Social Security Administration (SSA) programs organized to provide disability benefits for citizens unable to work. These benefits are granted under two separate programs: Social Security Disability Insurance (SSDI) and Supplemental Security Income (SSI). Benefits under SSDI are considered entitlements earned by contributing wage earners. SSI is a form of welfare payment available for indigent persons who are elderly or living with a disability. Enrollment in either program is contingent on a review of the individual's work history, medical opinion as to any disability and its effects, and a determination as to whether an individual has the mental and physical capacity to complete tasks associated with previous employment or to receive training for a new occupation.

The SSA maintains a list of nine psychiatric diagnostic categories that constitute impairments for which an applicant may seek benefits. Of these, the women interviewed for this study typically filed claims that fell within the categories of schizophrenia, paranoid and other psychotic disorders, mood disorders, anxiety-related disorders, and substance abuse disorders. For example, Marvella, who was diagnosed with both PTSD and schizophrenia by psychiatrists in Colorado, had received SSI while a resident of Denver. Upon moving to Los Angeles and thus switching states, she was required to reapply for benefits. This process entails going through a new series of assessments. "They have their own mental health doctor they want you to see," she explains. "I have yet to receive any of those dates or appointments. I would assume . . . my counselor over here told me they'd also be wanting his input for the assessments and stuff." Shawna was previously in a similar position. Having moved across several states, she is now in Los Angeles to pursue a career in the entertainment industry for her eight-year-old daughter. As a result of these moves, Shawna had had multiple experiences of filing SSI claims over the years. Her first claim, some eight years earlier, was based on the fact, she says, that she had "developmental issues all growing up. Like, I had learning disabilities, [and] I had mental problems." When Shawna is asked about her understanding of the claim process, she admits, "I don't even know. I still to this day . . . it's been eight years, and to this day I still don't know. All I know is I saw the doctor, and the next thing I know, I saw that I was approved." Having been repeatedly denied in Illinois, she is now again approved and receiving SSI benefits in California.

One of the primary conditions attached to receipt of SSI or SSDI benefits is compliance with prescribed treatment. The SSA's position is that failure to comply with any treatment deemed as offering the potential to improve functioning is a deliberate barrier to returning to work and thus grounds for denial or discontinuation of a claim (Leo and Del Regno 2001).[5] The practical effect of this rule is that women who apply for SSDI on mental health grounds are placed in the position of having to either follow prescribed drug treatment plans or pretend to comply in order to skirt the rule. Serafina is one of the former group. In response to a question about where she sees herself in the future, she replies, "In five years I hope my SSDI goes through [laughs], so I could get somewhere." She's presently living on about $200 a month and is eager to get out of the shelter. When queried about the status of her claim, she responds, "I'm just waiting for my pill for my disability." Jan is presently receiving "income from disability . . . 'cause I have rheumatoid arthritis and they say paranoid schizophrenic and all this stuff." Although Jan never openly states that she is flouting the SSA rules, as indicated in the previous chapter, she had discontinued using Prozac and refuses to take the antipsychotic drug quetiapine, which was prescribed to her.[6] Mercy, who has been repeatedly hospitalized for severe depression since the passing of her mother two years ago, is also cautious to never openly state that she too flouts the SSA rules.

LAURA: Has your psychiatrist told you to take any medications?
MERCY: Yeah.
LAURA: Are you taking anything?
MERCY: I get it.
LAURA: You get it, but do you take it?
MERCY: [silence][makes a face]
MERCY: [laughs] It doesn't do anything for me. I do it for the SSI.

Mercy then admits that, because her prescriptions for perphenazine and amitriptyline "don't do anything" in terms of lifting her depression or addressing her other mental and emotional issues, she doesn't take them. She makes, however, one exception: "I take [them] for four days before when they have to check my blood, but otherwise I don't." She also makes sure to pick up her prescriptions because her doctor checks, and she fears being reported to SSA for noncompliance and thus losing her benefits. "He has to tell them," she states, "because it's mental health." This same fear prompts Marilyn to comply with her psychiatrist's orders: "You gotta do what they tell you to do," Marilyn sighs, "[or] they will cut it off and it's hard to get back." Conversely, Donna, who is waiting for her SSDI claim to be approved, is openly vocal about her intention to break the treatment compliance rule: "I'm not going to take no pills. I'm gonna fake it, so that I can get my mental health. I can get my SSDI." Donna feels she is justified: "That's my money, [and] I'm going to get it." Should Donna be caught, she runs the risk of not only having her benefits terminated but, given that she was referred to the psychiatric service for "bumping heads," possibly being kicked out of the shelter. Donna is fortunate in that she is not staying at one of the shelters where staff members supervise med calls, having clients sign a register that records their daily drug intake. Were that the case, information regarding her lack of compliance could be shared with SSA officials.

Criminal Justice System

Many of the women who reside in Los Angeles shelters have experienced incarceration. Although most of these experiences were in police lockup or county jail, several participants were imprisoned in state correctional facilities. Several had their first experiences with mental health services and the use of psychiatric drugs while in state prison.

Tess's story is a case in point: her first exposure to the use of prescription psychoactive drugs occurred while she was serving a state prison sentence for auto theft. At first, she was in a state of shock over her arrest and trial. That shock quickly gave way to fear when the first-time offender received a two-year sentence: "I was really scared [of what would happen in prison] because I watch too much TV." She adds, "Here I am in prison, my first time ever being incarcerated, and I'm tripping out." Although she would only serve ten months of that two-year sentence, those months "felt like ten years." To help her pass the time more bearably, more experienced prisoners advised her to fake a mental health condition in order to get a prescription for a heavy sedative. "I said, 'I want to sleep my time away,' so we go get some meds . . . so that's what I did. I went and I was doped up. Wait here for dinner, wait here for lunch, and the next thing you know it's time to go home." To execute the plan, Tess presented herself to a prison psychiatrist as someone suffering from depression. At first she was prescribed the drugs venlafaxine and escitalopram, which did not have the desired effect. Coached by other prisoners, she then told the psychiatrist she had been taking quetiapine, an antipsychotic that has been used as a sleeping aid. "I wanted to sleep my time away, so I said, 'Hey, I'm taking meds on the outs,' because they don't check. You can go in the pen and say you took anything, and they're going to give it to you." She even asked for the quetiapine in a specific form because she had been told that "syrup, that's the medication to take in the pen and you'll sleep." She was placed on 800 milligrams of quetiapine a day. At first, her response to the drug was to tell the psychiatrist, "I need more. I need more." However, as I noted in the last chapter, Tess began to experience some of the drug's serious adverse metabolic side effects, including a significant weight gain. "I gotta get off this shit," she decided, because "that shit messes you up." Now fearing for her health, she returned to the prison psychiatrist and told the truth: "I told the prison I lied." Likely seeing this new admission as evidence of delusional behavior ("lack of insight"), the psychiatrist did not believe her. "He didn't want to hear it, so I just slept, and they didn't care."

Some of the women interviewed for this study were on probation at the time of their participation and residing in shelters as part of a California initiative known as AB109. In 2011, California governor Edmund Brown, Jr., signed into law Assembly Bills 109 and 117, which were intended to help resolve some of California's penal overcrowding problem by keeping nonserious "offenders" out of state prisons and off parole lists. Under AB109, these offenders, once released from county jail, would be supervised in the community by probation officers. A major component of this initiative is focused on the postrelease treatment of offenders identified as having mental health issues. To identify such individuals, staff from the Los Angeles County Department of Mental Health (LACDMH) are colocated with Probation Services at a prerelease center and tasked with screening individuals eligible for AB109 release and, through the use of prison medical records, identifying those diagnosed with mental health or substance abuse issues (Marx and McCravey 2012). Such individuals are subject to service needs assessments and are referred for appropriate treatment, with staff "work[ing] with [the] client to engage recommended treatment option" (Marx and McCravey 2012). Such treatment is said to be "voluntary"; however, acknowledge that treatment is actually a "condition of supervision" and that "sanctions by Probation for failure to comply" with treatment may result (Marx and McCravey 2012). To help ensure compliance, medication support programs are included among the postrelease services provided (Marx and McCravey 2012).

Joelle is one of the women on AB109 release. In prison, she had been diagnosed with anxiety and depression with psychotic features. One psychiatrist prescribed fluoxetine, telling her, "This is supposed to fix everything." When the drug had no effect, the blame was placed on Joelle. She was told "to start taking my medication more." Once released from prison, she was assigned a community-based psychiatrist, who changed her prescription to the antipsychotic drug aripiprazole. Aripiprazole also had no effect on her anxiety, and Joelle, a sexual abuse survivor, continued to have panic attacks. When she tried to explain her situation to the new psychiatrist, her concerns were dismissed in what she describes as a humiliating scene: "The one time I talked to him, the way he came off, he was just . . . what I was going through was bullshit to him. I sat there and teared up and . . . I got emotional and I was trying to explain to him about my medication and stuff . . . [stops speaking]." Despite Joelle's legitimate concerns about her mental health issues and the effects (or lack thereof) of the drug prescribed, the psychiatrist refused to alter the prescription. Had Joelle been in another set of circumstances, she would simply have fired the psychiatrist and sought treatment elsewhere. However, as a former prisoner on AB109 release, that option was not available to her. As a condition of release, she is forced to comply with the psychiatrist's directives or risk sanctions, which could include jeopardizing her release status. Angelique, who clearly states that enforcing treatment compliance simply will not work with her, is notably one of those women who has been on an AB109 release and has had her probation status revoked, necessitating a period in jail when she refused to comply with her probation conditions.

Inpatient Psychiatric Facilities

Another means by which psychiatric drug treatment is enforced is through admissions into a psychiatric facility. In some instances, admissions are voluntary, as occurred with Jan, who had sought inpatient treatment. In her own words, Jan says she "went to the psych ward" because she "had a nervous breakdown" following her ex-husband's arrest for murder: "I was clean and my NA [narcotics anonymous] sponsor, she said, 'Honey, you looked razzled. You need to go get some help. Get some time. Just go in.' It was a residential place, and they knew the people 'cause they worked in that field, and they sent me over there." It was at this time that Jan was placed on quetiapine, which she agreed to take because she believed that it would help her. Today, she feels that it is "a mild sedative" that "didn't really change anything." As if to provide evidence, she notes that following her release, she returned to the facility two further times in search of help: "I thought I was going crazy. I couldn't believe it." Alex finds the machines and the staff at the local hospitals soothing. Thus, whenever she feels the pressures of her life are too much to bear and she needs a respite, she presents herself at one of the local hospitals and asks to be admitted.

California state law also allows for involuntary confinement of individuals who are diagnosed with a "serious mental illness" and are deemed to be either gravely disabled or to pose a danger to themselves or others. Under Section 5150 of the California Welfare and Institutions Code, a police officer or clinician can place individuals under arrest for the purpose of transporting them to a psychiatric facility, where they can be held for up to seventy-two hours. Kerry is one of the women who have been arrested by the police as a "5150," as is Freda. Freda has been "5150'd" twice. She acknowledges that the first time the police were called, she was having "a paranoid episode." However, the second phone call came as a result of an ongoing dispute with neighbors: "They call 911. 'We got a 5150. 911, she's over here threatening to kill us or something.' They can take you on harm to yourself, harm to others. There's no questions asked. Or the more you get upset, the more it's like you are crazy. So you gotta go. They gotta check me out." Mercy, who fell into a deep depression following her mother's death that resulted in periods during which she wouldn't bathe or eat, doesn't recall the circumstances surrounding her first psychiatric confinement. Mercy's social worker subsequently informed her that she was placed under a 5150 hold because she was suicidal. Of this episode, she says, "I don't remember telling them that I wanted to hurt myself." Since this initial hospitalization, Mercy estimates she has "been in and out" of psych wards "like twelve times." Sometimes she presents herself to a clinician at her local mental health center knowing she will be "5150'd" and thus readmitted. Like Alex, Mercy forces her admission when she feels she needs a respite from the streets and her ongoing emotional and mental problems. She has also been "5150'd" after calling the police because she simply wanted "to have someone to talk to."

Once admitted, individuals are assessed in order to make a determination as to whether continued confinement is warranted. If individuals are deemed unfit for release, Section 5250 allows the initial seventy-two-hour period to be extended for up to fourteen days. One woman who has experienced the consequences of this law is Melanie, who has just been released from confinement following a mental health capacity hearing. "My last hospitalization was in July," she says. "They had me as 5250. I had to go to court to see the judge to claim my competency." She is grateful to be "back on the streets" and feels that "if the judge hadn't let me out, I'd probably been there for a year." This experience was not Melanie's first with involuntary commitment: "I suffer from schizophrenia, so I stay back and forth in the mental hospital." Whereas previous confinements had been at "hospitals here in Los Angeles, [where] they give you your regular meds and they don't really drug you out," her last involuntary stay had been at a facility where sedation was more heavily used. As a result she wanted to leave. To illustrate, she describes a place where the activities and behaviors of patients are carefully controlled through heavy sedation: "All they did was feed you full of meds, and you walk around like a bunch of cows all day grazing grass. They feed you and they med you and then they want you to do arts and crafts." Freda's experiences of involuntary admissions echo those of Melanie: "I hate going to those hospitals because you try to talk to them, and unfortunately most of the nurses are assholes. They're doing their job. Here's your pills, take 'em, [and] get away from me." The Pastor had also had one experience of involuntary admission, which followed a visit to a mental health center. She describes this experience as solidifying her belief that "drugs are a curse":

> You take the medicine, you're all out of it, then they put you in with mental patients, and if you keep on taking it, you be gone. . . . [A]t [the] hospital, they gave me so much medicine, and she was like, "You're going to have to take your medicine." I didn't want it, and the lady told me, "If you come back here, they're going to lock you up." I just sat there. I never said anything. I just waited for the doctor. Days went by and I said, "I'm still waiting for a doctor." I took one pill from two ladies, and my mind was just totally out of it. . . . I cried after that.

Although none of the women interviewed for this project spoke of having been subjected to this section of the Welfare and Institutions Code, Section 5334 allows superior court officials to make determinations as to whether an individual should be permitted to decline treatment with antipsychotic drugs. Individuals who are deemed to be lacking the capacity to make an informed choice on the matter can be given such drugs against their will for the duration of the time they are being held (Welfare and Institutions Code, s. 5336).

Community Mental Health Programs

Through local service providers, LACDMH operates a number of programs and services for homeless citizens with psychiatric diagnoses. Such programs variously include clinical outreach, mental health referral, housing, and service needs assessment components. The county also supports locally run "wellness centers," the purpose of which is to provide community-based support for "adult clients to assist them on the road to recovery from their mental illness" (LACDMH 2016). As evidenced in Hannah's story, among the services offered by wellness centers are medication support and prescription management programs (LACDMCH 2016). Monique is enrolled in one of these programs. Now fifty-five, Monique was first diagnosed with schizophrenia at the age of twenty-nine, some nine years after she was physically and sexually assaulted while on a date. Over the years, her original diagnosis was revised to schizoaffective disorder. Each month Monique goes to her local mental health center, where she receives a shot from a community nurse of paliperidone, a drug labeled as an antipsychotic treatment. For the remainder of the month, Monique attends weekly psychotherapy, as well as group classes, both of which stress the importance of treatment compliance. Of the drug injections, she says, "I do it because I want to get better." However, when asked if she feels the drug is helping her condition, she says it is not and that she continues to struggle with some of her fixed beliefs.[7]

Although Alex is presently staying at a shelter in Pasadena, she was previously enrolled in a med program in North County, in the San Diego area. Whereas in Pasadena Alex can simply take her prescriptions to be filled at a local pharmacy to be subsequently dispensed at her shelter's 7:00 PM med call, the North County program requires oversight and monitoring of psychiatric patients' treatment compliance. Alex explains: "They stand right there and watch you take it . . . [and] I have to go sit with the psychologist. We talk. She takes me to the room; the doctors are there. They have the uniform; they know what they're doing. They pull it out, and they say, 'Take it.'" Like Hannah, Alex was also enrolled in group classes aimed at fostering compliance. The "psycho class," as she calls it, was oriented toward explaining to participants "why the mind is telling me that I don't want to take [the prescribed drugs]." She continues, "Those classes, we're sitting in a group and they're explaining it, talking about it." Alex loved the classes because they provided her with a caring environment that has been otherwise lacking in her life:

> It's very supportive, the group. It's like, "I'm taking it. Are you taking your medication?" We have that support, that love, that care. So I'm not alone. I don't feel alone in taking the medication. We're doing it all as a group together. I like the environment. I like the groups. I participate. There's a lot of love, a lot of care for me. I feel well inside the group.

As is also the case with Hannah and Monique, Alex has internalized the group's dominant messages to a significant degree. As a result of having read up on the possible side effects of risperidone, she professes a fear of taking the drug but continues to take it: "Why wouldn't I take it if I need it to stay alive? I'm not going to do that to myself. I don't want to die or be in the mental hospital, so I take it."

California state law also provides a mechanism for courts to order individuals who refuse to comply with psychiatric drug treatment into "assisted outpatient treatment" (AOT). This process was implemented into law as the result of a California case in which a psychiatric patient, Scott Thorpe, walked into a mental health clinic in 2001 and began a shooting rampage that killed three people. In response, the parents of victim Laura Wilcox pushed California legislators for the passage of Assembly Bill 1421 (known as Laura's Law).[8] Laura's Law provides counties with the ability to use AOTs (also known as community treatment orders) as a means of enforcing treatment compliance in the community. For a citizen to be subject to the conditions of Laura's Law, the individual must

1. Be eighteen years of age or older.[9]
2. Have been diagnosed with a "serious mental disorder."
3. Have a history of treatment noncompliance.
4. Have refused offers of community-based treatment.
5. Have been determined to be "at-risk" in the community without supervision.
6. Have a condition that is believed to be deteriorating.

The term *serious mental disorder* is defined in the bill as any disorder appearing in the current edition of DSM, with the exception of developmental disorders, traumatic brain injuries, and substance use disorders. To guide courts on the issue of whether an individual has a history of treatment compliance, factors to be considered include whether the person has had two or more hospitalizations or periods of incarceration within the previous three years, or whether the individual has threatened or committed one or more acts of serious violence to himself or herself or others. The bill also identifies specific "target populations," members of which might be more likely to require "outreach and treatment options." One of these groups is "homeless persons who are mentally ill" (California Code, s. 5600.3).

Citing a lack of funds to support AOT programs, Los Angeles County implemented Laura's Law in 2010 on a limited basis. As a result, the number of individuals in Los Angeles County placed in an AOT program has been low: in the first year of its implementation, eighteen individuals in the county were ordered into an AOT program (Fujioka 2012). Despite limited use of the legislation, when Laura's Law was due to sunset in January 2013. Los Angeles County officials, among other counties, lobbied state legislators in support of a new bill (AB1569) that would extend Laura's Law to 2019 (Fujioka 2012). They also asked for increased state funding to expand AOT within their county (Fujioka 2012). State officials responded to these pleas by passing the new bill and providing individual counties with the ability to divert funds available to them under the Mental Health Services Act to support AOT programs. In response, in 2014 Los Angeles County began preparing plans to fully implement Laura's Law (Esquivel 2014). These plans include the development of an AOT team that will "screen requests, conduct extensive outreach and engagement, develop petitions and manage the court processes to connect AOT enrollees with [existing] service providers" (LACDMH 2013). Although not fully operational at the time of writing, and thus not directly relevant to the current treatment of the women in this study, the law, once fully implemented, will result in a number of homeless women within the county inevitably finding themselves subject to enforced psychiatric treatment in the community. One official who was queried about Laura's Law estimated that by 2015 the number of individuals within the Los Angeles program would increase to approximately 300. As to the ultimate utility of this law, that issue remains debatable. When Kerry and Angelique, two women with years of experience with homelessness and the mental health system, are asked for their thoughts on Laura's Law, they both scoff at the idea that this measure would be useful for helping them or others to deal with their issues. Angelique is particularly emphatic in her views: "I take my meds because I choose to." Any attempt at enforcing compliance, she says, "won't work for me." To illustrate her point, Angelique estimates that she has been "5150'd" some sixteen times and is now compliant because she chooses to be.

Freda shares Angelique's views on the issue of community treatment orders. Describing what that experience of an involuntary hold and forced treatment feels like for the individual, Freda, who is herself treatment compliant by choice, says the system simply makes people "feel like they've got no control." To illustrate this point, she notes that individuals are dehumanized or pathologized in ways that make them feel less than worthy of respect or consideration. Referring to inpatient staff, she says, "It's hard to communicate with them because they already see you as in a psychosis or something." Because Freda sees patient disempowerment as counterproductive to healing, like Angelique, she disagrees with the idea of the state creating and using more tools to force people into complying with psychiatric orders. What has worked for Freda, according to Freda, is not strategies of control that lead to her further disempowerment—she is, after all, an impoverished, homosexual, African American woman (i.e., a victim of structural violence) diagnosed with a stigmatizing psychiatric disorder—but rather therapeutic techniques that she finds self-empowering. For example, as first explained in Chapter 4, Freda credits her attendance at local college courses with allowing her to develop insights into her functioning and to learn tools that she practices on a daily basis:

> How I deal with it is self-talk. The best thing is when I went to college and took psychology. I went to learn about my disorder. I learned self-talk. Reminding yourself that I have a mental disorder. This may or may

> not be true. The nurse is just watching me. She just happened to say something I was thinking about. It doesn't mean you can read people's minds. You can get caught up in it, so I do self-talk. But not like walking down the street, "I'm going to do this, that." [Laughs.] People think you're crazy; you're talking to yourself. [Laughs.] You just remind yourself that you have a disorder. I remind myself that thing that I'm worrying about doesn't exist.

Tools learned from her course work are complemented by other coping strategies that Freda has received through working intensively with a therapist. We note that she seems to be "working a good program," and her agreement reveals some of that insight: "I do, but like every human, I get complacent, so I could use the coping skills of being assertive and not aggressive. Sometimes it's human nature. You want to act out. So I've got to stay a little focused, continuing with the coping skills. I realized I can't stop. I'll get the coping skills and all that information, and I'll think I'm cured, and I'm not. I've got to keep going."

Hard or Soft: Does It Matter?

Within homeless communities, institutions play a valuable role in promoting treatment compliance. Indeed, as must be acknowledged, the original purpose behind early testing of chlorpromazine was to establish its effectiveness in treating manic symptoms among hospitalized psychiatric patients—in other words, to find a means of rendering a portion of a marginalized population more manageable within the confines of the institution within which they were housed. Although seemingly more people in the general population have been turning to psychiatric drugs in order to smooth out the rough edges of their lives, or as part of an ethics of self-care aimed at enhancing one's "neurochemical self" (Rose 2003), the use of psychiatric drugs within marginalized communities resembles more closely their earlier use within institutions. We are not suggesting that the two are mutually exclusive; indeed, within homeless communities, these are often complementary processes to achieving treatment compliance.

Soft forms of compliance-oriented techniques, found principally within community settings such as shelters and mental health centers, operate primarily, but not solely, through persuasion. For example, group therapy classes at local mental health centers attempt to create something many of the women interviewed have lacked from the beginning of their lives: a nurturing, supportive environment. Alex, who was bullied by her father for her sexual identity and sexually molested by an unnamed family member, takes great comfort from the support she receives at the group therapy sessions at her local center, sessions that mingle expressions of love and empathy with pro–drug treatment messages. On the surface, this caring environment provides Alex with the emotional nourishment she clearly craves. However, it has its own subtly coercive edge: this love is not unconditional. Instead, a lingering, implicit threat always lingers that such support can be withdrawn from the recalcitrant. Further, clinicians at wellness centers are invested with the power to sanction noncompliant individuals through a range of actions, from reporting them to the SSA for noncompliance, to involuntary confinement, and, soon, to engaging in forcible treatment of the noncompliant within the community through an AOT.[10] Shelters, which run such apparently benign programs such as med calls, both supervise and monitor individuals' drug-taking practices. And, not coincidentally, individuals who are seen by case managers as engaging in problematic behaviors, as is the case with Donna, are referred to psychiatric treatment and told they need "meds."[11] The threat hanging over Donna's head, and the heads of countless other women, is that unwillingness to comply with psychiatric treatment and mend their behaviors will result in their being "turned out" of the facility or difficulties with receiving income support through disability programs. We view such threats as problematic given the tendency observed is that women use psychiatric drugs as their only form of treatment when, in many instances, women also appeared to need other more comprehensive therapeutic approaches that would also allow them to begin the process of addressing unresolved trauma, the effects of structural violence, and other underlying issues.[12]

The experiences of women who have been confronted by the harder, more coercive edge of the mental health system illustrate the roles that institutions can play in forcibly garnering compliance, from inpatient facilities to the criminal justice system. What these experiences also reveal is that coercion does not always work. The fact that Angelique, Kerry, Joelle, Freda, Melanie, Mercy, and countless others have been existing within a cycle of involuntary confinements, from jails to locked hospital wards, would seem to offer support for this claim. Of these particular six women, four—Angelique, Joelle, Kerry, and Freda—state they have made the conscious choice to follow their prescribed drug treatments. And only one, Freda, seems to be making progress in her attempts at addressing her current situation, though, for this development, Freda credits "self-talk" and "coping tools" and not psychiatric drugs or involuntary confinement. In this regard, Freda is not dissimilar to women like Deborah and Kathy, whose stories were shared in the last chapter. Of the other compliant women listed above, Joelle is struggling and appears to only be following the prescribed treatment program because she is currently on probation and fears returning to jail. Kerry, as reported elsewhere, is smoking crack. Angelique, a victim of years of sexual abuse within her family and the foster care system, maintains a difficult relationship with the psychiatric drugs she has been taking, being at one point so heavily sedated that she passed out at her mental health center. At various times, she has stopped taking them and likely will do so again in the future. One should remember that, to the extent they are presently treatment compliant, these are individuals who represent institutional success stories.

Other women who similarly represent the so-called success of procompliance measures are faring no better. Although Monique, Alex, and Hannah are each treatment compliant, and none are presently in either jail or a psychiatric facility, all have been homeless for years. Further, Monique acknowledges that her "med" has no effect on her beliefs, Alex uses inpatient services as a sanctuary, and Hannah's alogia, among other signs, evidences the reality that the drugs prescribed for her do not, nor can they, effectively treat her underlying condition. All of this raises an interesting question: What's the point?

Notes

1. A search of online forums confirms that side effects reported by risperidone users include feeling pressure in the ears, hearing the sound of fluids in the ear canal, and experiencing ringing (tinnitus).

2. A possible diversion program that may be available to women dealing with addiction would be sober-living homes (see http://soberliving.interventionamerica.org/). These facilities serve as a "boundary institution" in the management of poverty (see Fairbanks 2009 for additional information).

3. We must acknowledge here that the case manager is also likely trying to keep Donna and other residents safe in light of Donna's aggressive tendencies.

4. In terms of compliance, however, we saw no evidence of peer pressure and peer surveillance.

5. In 2009 the US Eighth Circuit Court of Appeals carved out an exception for individuals diagnosed with one of the SSA's enumerated mental health conditions: if evidence can be produced that failure to follow prescribed treatment is a symptom of the condition, a determination primarily based on psychiatric report, the claim can proceed or the individual will continue to receive help (see *Pate-Fires v. Astrue*, 564 F.3d 935 [8th Cir. 2009]). The reality is, of course, that many homeless citizens would either be unaware of this exception, nor would most have the means to assert their rights under law.

6. Given Jan's diagnosis, however, her case would likely fall within the exception carved out by the *Pate-Fires* case cited in note 5 above.

7. Although she openly frames one of her delusory beliefs as a product of her psychiatric condition, Monique still remains hopeful that she will one day marry the rapper Sean "P. Diddy" Combs.

8. Laura's Law is modeled on a similar bill in New York (Kendra's Law). California and New York are only two of forty-four states that have some form of legislation allowing applications to be made to the courts to force individuals into treatment compliance within the community (Appelbaum 2003).

9. Adults are subject to Section 5600 of the code, whereas minors fall within the parameters of Section 5585.

10. We do not discount that positive work is also performed at shelters.

11. When we ran into Donna at the same shelter some nine months after her initial interview, she revealed that she has, indeed, gone to see the recommended psychiatrist and been given "psych medicine," which, true to her word, she has been secretly refusing to take.

12. We also recognize, again, that in some cases forced compliance may be necessary if an individual may be at significant risk of harm or of being harmful to others.

7

Changing the Status Quo

The seed for this book is planted when Laura is sitting in a doctor's office in a shelter, trying to catch up on notes from the previous interview before the next research participant walks in. A woman appears in the doorway, shuffles in slowly, and sits down. Betty is an African American woman; she is overweight and appears to be in her late fifties. Her age is difficult to guess because life on the streets takes a hard toll on the body. She is missing teeth, often a sign of advanced age, but here, in this shelter on the city's south side, it could also be the result of poor nutrition, inadequate dental care, drug use, or violence, or any combination thereof. But her teeth are not what has garnered Laura's attention; it's her tongue. As she silently listens to an explanation of the study, the woman's tongue repeatedly snakes in and out of her mouth. Throughout the course of the interview, this serpentine movement happens over and over again.

Upon seeing involuntary tics, shuffling gaits, and various odd physical movements, it is not unusual for people to assume these are, in and of themselves, signs of some serious disorder. But what Laura is observing, and would come to be seen in various guises over the next few years, is not the effects of a disease but those produced by the treatment. Betty has classic signs of iatrogenic neurological damage. In her case, the odd movements of her tongue are evidence of tardive dyskinesia, a movement disorder of the voluntary muscles, which is a side effect of some psychiatric drugs, typically those referred to as "antipsychotics" (Sethi 2004). As is the case with almost all of the women interviewed, Betty has experienced violence and abuse and has had an incredibly difficult life filled with enormous challenges. In every sense, she is a trauma survivor. And, like many other trauma survivors found within shelters, Betty's traumatic experiences have manifested in a collection of thoughts and behaviors that are seen as amenable to treatment with psychiatric drugs, drugs that can have as a side effect neurological damage (Demler 2014; Haddad and Dursun 2008).

Betty's experience with mental health treatment is very different from that of Lea, who resides in a women's shelter in Los Angeles's Skid Row District. Lea is a fifty-three-year-old recovering alcoholic and drug addict whose addictions began with her son's death in 2008. As her life began to rapidly spiral downward, she lost custody of her remaining children. After being adrift for a year, Lea met a man, fell in love, and began the process of rebuilding her life. Two weeks before they were to be married, Lea's fiancé was killed in a workplace accident. She fell back into her addictions, became homeless, and began engaging in sex work to survive. Seeking help, Lea had come to the shelter, where her case manager placed her in various addiction support programs and into individual sessions with a psychotherapist who had been trained in trauma-informed therapy. Understanding that the root of Lea's problems was the grief she was feeling over the loss of two of the most important people in her life, the therapist devised a plan. Lea explains:

> She brought me a little box and on the outside of the box it had all the things that make me want to go forward, and inside of the box were the things that held me back, which were the deaths. So I had pictures of my son, I had pictures of my son's funeral, I had my fiancé's stuff in there, and knowing that I have to open it up sometime and pull something out to deal with it, to go forward, I would do that, and put my picture back in and seal the box because it had Velcro on it. All around it was my grandkids, my kids, my dad. So that's what helped me move forward. My therapist, she helped me through it.

Reflecting on the therapy process, Lea adds:

> My main thing when I came in here is that . . . I was broken . . . I was a broken person. Broken and lost. I needed help. I self-medicated so that I didn't deal with it, but I knew there would come a day that I needed to deal with it. The only thing I can say that really helped me . . . when I started here with my therapist . . . I didn't want to come back. After the first couple of times I came, I was like, "She's just hearing me out. She's not telling me what to do. She's just letting me talk." I wanted somebody to help me to cope with it. Then when she brought in this box, this box really helped me . . . that's what helped me … [and] after I got this box, I started looking forward to coming to my therapy sessions, because she'd be talking to me while I'd be pasting pictures. Little sayings that would come out of magazines. She brought me a whole stack of magazines; I just took letters and made words. Different things. That was my therapy.

Lea's experience reveals two key factors about healing and survival. First, like all women in our study, Lea needed to be heard by someone ready to hear her. She needed to find her voice and tell her story as part of her healing. Indeed, her therapist buying a "whole stack of magazines" appears to have been a remarkable gesture toward Lea. Not only did she note the gesture, but it clearly played a role in her healing processes (beyond enabling her to decorate and give meaning to her box): she felt someone cared and heard her. Second, it was the trauma-informed care, not simply the isolated use of chemicals, that enabled Lea to find a way to cope with her traumatic experiences. Lea, rather than suppress her pain through sedating prescription drugs, learned how to feel her pain, "deal with it," and move on.

Lea's experiences, in essence, highlight key realities that shape this final chapter. Specifically, we have two goals. The first is to provide a review of the key findings presented in order to bring our central argument to its final conclusion. That conclusion is simple: with the monopoly of the biopsychiatric model (the use of chemicals without therapy) within and across the institutions that structure homeless lives, highly traumatized individuals are essentially left untreated, their symptoms, too often, simply masked by psychiatric drugs. Although the manifestations of their emotional and other problems may no longer represent behavioral and other challenges for those institutions, for the individual carrying the burden of untreated trauma, nothing really changes. As a result, we can reasonably expect many of these citizens to continue to cycle in and out of homelessness, hospitals, jails, and other institutions.

Our second goal in this chapter is to offer an alternative to this exclusive reliance on psychiatric drugs by suggesting biopsych's failed chemical solutions be replaced with something that is significantly more likely to work with trauma survivors: trauma-informed therapy. What we argue in the final pages is that trauma-informed therapies, when combined with housing and social supports, represent means of engendering self-empowerment, by encouraging the ability of individuals to develop and use the tools they need to address the roots and manifestations of their distress.

Cuts, Chemicals, and Medicalization

We will begin with the undeniable trend that is medicalization, where treatments for normal life realities are now the norm, including the social truths surrounding homelessness and, most definitely, mental health.[1] Indeed, the DSM-V has been openly criticized for contributing to the medicalization of mental health (see Pickersgill 2013). Further, mental health has been redefined as a social problem that is psychiatric in origin, within a larger social framework that increasingly views the biopsychiatric worldview as providing the solution to most, if not all, of our complex and mundane problems. As such, one can easily see why biopsychiatry has been touted as the solution to homelessness, and unstinting faith has been placed in the chemical regimens often prescribed. This unwavering faith has had important consequences for how homeless citizens are treated. It has spawned new ways of thinking about and responding to their problems, which, on the surface, appear similar to how the problems of other segments of the population are viewed. Invoking a disease metaphor to explain the causes of their distress, homeless citizens learn their only hope is to participate in the treatment of their chemical imbalances—clearly medicalization in practice! Within this framework, responsibilized self-care is couched as an individually empowering act; however, as we shall discuss, it is ultimately one that does little more than maintain social and structural inequities that disempower the individuals most in need of help.

Further, psychiatric drugs are not therapeutic in the sense conventionally suggested; they do not return individuals to what others might see as a normal state of functioning. Indeed, the normal state for many of the individuals who find themselves being prescribed psychiatric drugs is the very state being chemically altered. Admittedly, as suggested in Chapter 3, *normal* is something of a loaded word in this discussion, as it more usually signifies some standard of behavior that the homeless are measured against when determining the type and degree of their purported pathology. However, when we say their behavior is normal in the present context, we are referring to the fact that the feelings, thoughts, and behaviors exhibited by the women we interviewed are not unusual for someone who has experienced significant trauma. As one of the authors, Laura, has been frequently heard to say, "You're normal for what you've been through."

So, if psychoactive drugs do not restore normal functioning, how then do neurochemicals work on the body of the individual, and, in particular, how do they work in ways that assist in the task of reforming the individual or modifying behaviors? The short answer is that they are shown to change the chemistry of the brain so as to place the individual into an altered state, which can have significant effects on mood, perception, cognition, speech, and behavior. Thus, leaving aside the possibility of placebo effects, as Joanna Moncrieff notes, when neurochemical treatments "work, or appear to work when they do, by putting people into a drug-induced state which is preferable (often to relatives and professionals, if not the person themselves) to whatever state they are in when drug-free" (2011, p. 175). With the drugs provided, homeless citizens often state that frequently the sedative properties of the drug produce beneficial effects.

As is known, traumatic events and other major life stressors, which in the case of homeless citizens are often chronic in nature, place tremendous pressure on individuals, particularly when they have few resources to draw upon. The result of these stressors is frequently the various signs of distress that are commonly seen in traumatized individuals treated for anxiety disorders, PTSD, major depression, BPD, and schizophrenia. Indeed, we are not discounting these diagnoses, and we further recognize that, when done properly, such diagnoses are made based on both clinical training and evidence and that psychiatric drugs would have the ability to reduce symptoms for such conditions—that is, *when* they do have an effect. If, for example, accepting that schizophrenia or PTSD is affected by, if not a direct product of, trauma and significant stressors, then of course these drugs will have a positive (and needed) effect. For example, sedation significantly impairs the individual's ability to fully experience painful feelings, which can help people learn to manage such feelings. Conversely, however, if a woman is depressed because she has lost her housing and is now living a precarious existence, a drug that purports to elevate her mood can potentially bring temporary relief. But the fact that such symptoms of distress abate does not mean the drugs are treating the symptoms of an underlying pathology, unless of course that pathological state is otherwise known as "poverty," "violence," "neglect," "lack of caring," or any one of a number of other adverse conditions of structural violence that women who are homeless face.

Notably, most women in our study are victims of structural violence: that is, violence embedded in a host of social, historical, and political forces that, directly or indirectly, perpetuate hardship by normalizing oppressive systems in societies (Bourgois, Prince, and Moss 2004; Farmer 2004, 2009; Hodgetts et al. 2014; Zizek 2008). These women are disempowered and largely unable to resist the powers of medical authorities who prescribe. Nonetheless, as Andrew Scull (2011) has suggested, the importance of symptom abatement for those individuals who are suffering should not be criticized. We understand this point. However, although, for some traumatized individuals, symptom abatement provides relief and is thus useful—that is, when it is combined with both the personal and social resources upon which the individual can draw to foster resiliency—sedation or the real or perceived effects of minor mood elevation are not sufficient alone to heal the mental and emotional wounds of trauma. The particularly troubling thing is that every day in clinical offices across the United States, doctors provide neurochemical solutions, and too often these prescriptions are not coupled with counseling or other forms of treatment. The consequences of administering psychiatric drugs to individuals with untreated trauma and few, if any, coping skills are worthy of concern, given these drugs do not cure either the ascribed underlying condition (i.e., any purported biological defect within the brain) or the actual problem (i.e., the untreated effects of traumatic experience). Nor do they even purport to.

Further, as evidenced in cases like those surrounding the Paxil lawsuits as noted in Chapter 1, such drugs can inflict serious harm on people who are already suffering. This harm comes in the form of some fairly debilitating side effects: addiction, significant metabolic changes, loss of sexual desire, and neuroleptic-induced damage, plus a host of other possible adverse reactions including increases in suicidal ideations among youth (Bentall 2009; Breggin 1991; Choong et al. 2012; Davis and Rosenbloom 2006; Fuller Torrey 2006; Holt and Peveler 2011; Llorente and Urrutia 2006; Moncreiff 2013; Reilly et al. 2000; Reynolds and Kirk 2010; Trollor, Chen, and Sachdev 2009; Watanabe, Suzuki, and Someya. 2013). Certainly, among the women interviewed for our study, we see evidence of this fact in the stories of Betty, Tess, and others.

Use of such drugs also comes with an increased risk of (re)victimization within a segment of the population that is already disproportionately victimized by violence (Browne and Bassuk 1997; Jasinski et al. 2010). Providing women with often highly sedating drugs that impair their psychomotor functioning, particularly when they live in the streets or in other communal spaces within which they are highly exposed and thus vulnerable, places them at a greater risk of physical and sexual assault. Here one can see how structural violence underpins instances where people who fail to sustain themselves and families or meet the current standards of self-reliance are met with punitive responses (Hodgetts et al. 2014). The women in this study, like Mercy, recognized and attempted to avert both the long-term side effects and the increased risk of victimization by not taking the medication, even at the risk of being sanctioned by one or more of the various institutions upon which they rely for income, food, and shelter.

The Proof and the Pudding

For researchers interested in the phenomenon of homelessness, the real test of whether something actually works is whether individuals become stably housed postintervention and then remain so. In other words, women who had psychiatric care under the biopsych model should not be experiencing multiple or prolonged periods of homelessness, but they clearly are. We need not quote statistics or cite individual stories to demonstrate how biopsychiatric solutions have fallen short in addressing the root causes of homelessness. This fact is abundantly manifest throughout the streets of Los Angeles and in other cities across the United States and North America. This inadequacy has tended to be obscured behind a series of victim-blaming strategies that paint suffering individuals as treatment noncompliant and their so-called diseases as treatment resistant. Instead, people living in poverty are stigmatized, and, by holding them personally responsible for their position, the lesser treatment of groups of individuals and the minimal support provided to them can be condoned by the government, making evident that structural violence is again at play (Hodgetts et al. 2014). We should note here that, just as Philippe Bourgois and his colleagues (2004) explain, beyond victim blaming, the lived experiences of marginalized and vulnerable populations are often seen as a consequence of self-destructive behaviors rather than any underlying structural factors. Our study clearly demonstrates how structural violence is omnipresent yet maintains its invisibility; it affects people marginalized by geography, class, and race and gender (see Farmer 2009). Women living on the streets enduring hardships are one of these marginalized, thus invisible, subpopulations.

Throughout this book, we focused on the three principal powers we see exercised in relation to the treatment of trauma survivors within the biopsych paradigm: those of diagnosis, prescription, and compliance. We pondered whether on their own each might produce beneficial effects for individuals that result in improvements in the quality of their lives. Certainly, we have been repeatedly presented with the idea that the very act of diagnosing someone with a psychiatric condition is helpful in that such diagnosis affords individuals insight into their problems and lessens the burden of stigma: "I'm not a bad person. I have a disease." Leaving aside the fact that redefining trauma as an incurable disease is fraught with real and potential adverse effects for many people, we think examining specific cases is instructive to see if diagnosis furnished insights that led to changes that improved women's situations. In the examples provided by Deborah and Kathy, both women actively embraced their diagnoses and credited the diagnostic process with generating self-understanding and positive personal change. However, we also have the example of Grace, who was diagnosed as bipolar in a psychiatric facility in 2012 and firmly believes her problems are neurochemical in nature. She speaks knowledgeably about her "chemical imbalance," even identifying specific neurotransmitters deemed responsible for the problems that have manifested in her life. Whereas Deborah and Kathy report positive growth that, in Deborah's case, has led to a positive housing outcome, the opposite has occurred for Grace. Not long after her diagnosis and inpatient treatment, Grace decided to abandon a somewhat precarious but housed existence in Las Vegas to move to Los Angeles with her abusive husband, a decision that precipitated her homelessness. Grace's housing problems, though, may be resolved in an unusual fashion: within the three months in which she has been living in Los Angeles, she has dumped her husband and, although still married, is now engaged to a new man she met at a local shelter.

One can reasonably and justly argue that diagnosis alone cannot be the sole factor in effecting positive changes, whether in relation to generating feelings of wellness or in creating positive employment or housing outcomes. Certainly, most people would agree that diagnosis is only a small part of the equation, and that benefits really reside in treatment, and thus treatment must also be considered. Turning to the power of prescription, in theory, individuals who have been taking prescribed psychiatric drug treatments for a period of six weeks or longer should not be numbered among those experiencing prolonged or multiple episodes of homelessness. Why? Because, in theory, after having their purported chemical imbalances addressed through psychiatric drugs, which supposedly restore their neurochemicals to a balanced state and thus abate their symptoms, they should be newly restored to normal health and in sufficient shape to begin the process of transitioning out of homelessness. And yet that is not what we see: a number of the participants in this study had been on psychiatric drugs for months and years and had either remained homeless for a prolonged period of time or were on a second, third, or fourth cycle of being homeless. Marvella is a case in point: now fifty-four, and having spent years taking numerous psychiatric drugs, she is presently on antidepressants and can only recall one three-year period in her adult years in which she had stable housing and employment.

Prescription alone then is clearly insufficient. There is, of course, the issue of treatment compliance, which has been raised as a reason why individuals deemed mentally ill have failed to become stably housed and employed (Dixon, Friedman, and Lehman 1993). In garnering that compliance, we see biopsych wielding its power—power that comes as a result of its access to social, political, legal, and cultural forms of capital and is embedded in structural and systemic violence—through a network of interinstitutional alliances. But does compliance itself, in any of its soft or hard forms, help to produce positive outcomes for the individual? Hannah's story is instructive here. As we know, she spent almost four years in an outpatient treatment program that was aimed at *persuading* her to become responsible for managing her illness, a responsibility that she has faithfully accepted. Despite her participation in the program, her continuing psychiatric care, and her compliance with the regimen of antipsychotic drugs prescribed for her, she has cycled in and out of homelessness, returning multiple times to the same shelter in Skid Row in which she was first encountered. The same is true of Alex, who is fairly firm in her belief that the psychiatric drugs she takes are keeping her alive. And yet these same drugs are not preventing her from being homeless or assisting her in any tangible way in getting her life on some sort of track that will aid her in exiting homelessness.

It is something of a depressing fact that a majority of the women interviewed for this project have experienced not only multiple traumatic events but also multiple episodes of homelessness. Some have had brief stints of being housed; others have had long periods of stability intermixed with episodes of couch surfing with friends and family, staying in shelters, or sleeping in tents or in cars. And for every story we hear about someone striving to finally break this cycle, a woman is encountered who has remained stuck for months, years, and even decades. Indeed, when Laura returned to one shelter after a nine-month absence, many of the women previously interviewed—individuals who had every intention of transitioning into permanent housing, employment, and better lives—were still there. They were stuck, still seeing their psychiatrists, still taking their prescriptions, and still planning on getting out someday. They include women like Elise, who has been through nearly every type of biopsychiatric treatment in vogue since the 1970s, and who tells me in a highly thoughtful and lucid manner that she does not want to spend her final years in a shelter or dying in a park.

The reason often suggested for individuals' inability to escape homelessness permanently is that they are mentally ill, and that mental illness is a lifelong disease from which one rarely, if ever, recovers. Thus, proponents of this model assert the view that biopsychiatry is not at fault even though the majority of women in a state of homelessness who use its products never demonstrate substantial improvements in their overall health and well-being. Nor is biopsychiatry at fault because they tend not to find stable, let alone gainful, employment or remain in permanent housing. The fault lies with the individuals' biochemistry or the way the disease has manifested in their bodies that leaves women trapped in such cycles of homelessness. In support of this view, the diagnosis of schizophrenia is used as the example par excellence of the intractable mental illness. Leaving aside the fact of spontaneous remission and recovery in diagnosed schizophrenia cases (Andreason et al. 2005), schizophrenia, although overrepresented in homeless communities relative to diagnosis rates within the general population (Robertson and Winkleby 1996), still remains a less frequently diagnosed condition among homeless women when compared to higher rates of depression and anxiety and anxiety-related conditions (Bassuk et al. 1998;

Greifenhagen and Fichter 1997). So, in essence, proponents of the argument that the intractability of mental illness leads to a cycling in and out of homelessness are either using a minority of cases to define "mental illness" to make the broader case for how society ought to understand the lives of homeless women or else arguing that anxiety and depression, which are clearly tied to situational factors in the instant cases, are also intractable conditions akin to schizophrenia. The most manifest evidence of this line of thought comes in the form of the lists and pill bottles women carry, which reveal the types and volumes of psychiatric drugs being dispensed to them. What is evidenced, as documented in Chapter 4, is how frequently women are being prescribed a barrage of sedating drugs. Thus, these individuals who are already struggling to cope with multiple difficulties—always victims of structural violence—are having to do so under the additional burden of being sedated.

Why Do such Prescribing Practices Continue?

If psychiatric drugs in isolation, without counseling and other treatment, appear not to have significant long-term beneficial effects on the well-being and functioning of those treated with them, why do such prescribing practices continue to be used with homeless citizens? In the case of members of society at large, the partial answer was provided in Chapter 2: we as a society have adopted an ideological worldview that holds scientific studies in positions of dominance given they are believed to always produce superior knowledge.[2] For instance, if the results of a random control trial say that Drug X is, statistically speaking, more effective than a placebo, then Drug X must work. And if that drug works, the cause of the underlying condition must be biochemical in nature. Of course, we are assisted in our beliefs both by a barrage of scientists making strong claims to this effect and by uncritical mass media hype and pharmaceutical advertising on such topics as "the science of depression."[3]

In the case of the psychiatric treatment of homeless citizens, at least two immediate answers come to mind. First, the dominant worldview compels one to see social and individual problems through the lens of biopsychiatry, encouraging the treatment of social issues related to homelessness as biopsychiatric problems that require biopsychiatric solutions. In this sense, the treatment of homeless citizens is no different than the treatment of members of other social groups, too often with an exclusive reliance on pills to make someone feel better. Second, drugs are cheaper than quality therapy, which takes the time and skill of highly trained clinicians and requires the willingness of insurers and taxpayers to bear the cost. The profit logic that animates modern societies conditions citizens to hate investing in policies and programs that only pay out in the long term, particularly when the belief is put forth by some that a cheap, quick fix is available. Certainly, sedating individuals who might otherwise be problematic to deal with along with convincing others that a depression pill will lift their moods and make them feel better about their terrible situation are perfect examples of the types of quick fixes public policy makers and institutions with budget constraints may pin their hopes on.

What an Alternate Universe Might Look Like

Thus far, we have spent a great number of pages discussing what appears *not* to work in addressing the mental, emotional, and physical distress that frequently define the condition of homelessness. In this section we would like to draw on the data collected, the relevant research literature, and observations in the field to suggest a more fruitful approach, one that is focused on empowering rather than sedating individuals. Further, we want to reiterate that we recognize no credible position in psychiatry holds the expectation that psychotropic medical treatment alone would return individuals to

Photo 7.1 Unintentional Irony? Sign Posted in a Shelter Office

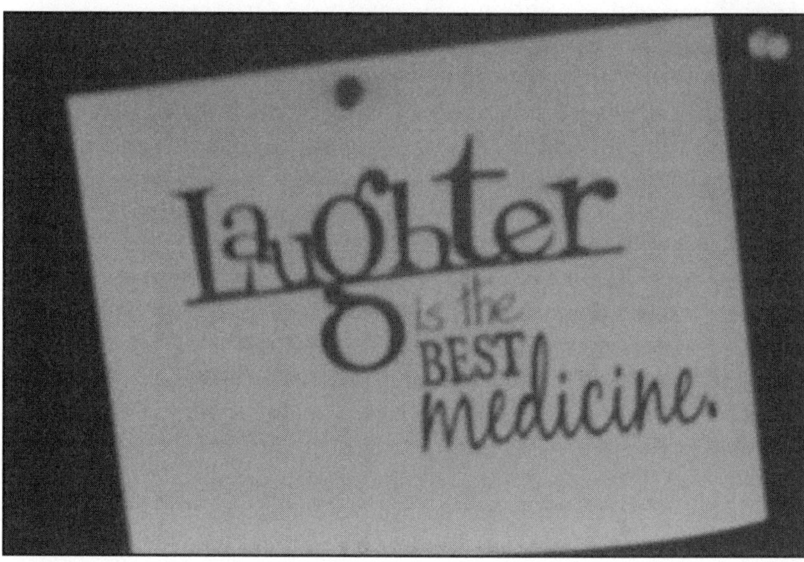

their normal state of functioning; however, we do recognize that too often such drugs are prescribed in isolation as treatment, in particular by many in the United States (in this case California) who have the power to prescribe. And this reality is what we take issue with. As such, our advocated approach entails the provision of three key, interrelated components: trauma-informed therapy, stable housing, and positive social networks.

Throughout some of the preceding chapters, we discussed or referenced the use of psychological or counseling services, often in the context of discussions on the types of services women accessed through their local mental health centers and their feelings about the utility of different forms of treatment. Reflecting on the thoughts and experiences shared in this area, we find most readily apparent is that what most women truly wanted, and several said so explicitly, was quality therapeutic counseling of the type described by Lea: empowering, empathic, and coconstructed, delivering lasting tools and insights that women could employ to manage symptoms of distress that could and would arise in their daily lives. Elsewhere, failures in the provision of quality psychological services to impoverished women in need are documented (Huey, Fthenos, and Hryniewicz 2012). Many of the same problems detailed in this earlier work were also seen in the experiences of the women interviewed for this project, from problems accessing services to counseling interns cycling in and out of programs to cuts to services.[4] However, in Los Angeles, some women, such as Lea, were receiving quality therapy and others, like Freda, had access to information and resources they could then use to aid in their own self-development. What the various forms of therapeutic dynamics, tools, and strategies referenced by these women share is that they typically came from, or were aligned with, a perspective that explicitly recognizes the fact that these women, as individuals, are suffering from the aftereffects of traumatic experiences. Without such recognition and intensive healing work in this area of their lives, this trauma remains unhealed and individuals remain stuck in the maladaptive patterns and negative coping strategies that keep too many trapped in homelessness and in cycles of institutionalization.

In essence, then, what we are suggesting is a move away from isolated treatment through pharmacology and instead toward the adoption of programs based on trauma-informed care. We do not wish to set up an artificial duality between these two modes of treatment, as we recognize that nothing is inherent to trauma-informed care that would preclude the use of psychotropic medication. What we are referring to is a set of therapeutic approaches that operate according to certain key principles. Among these is the adoption of a strength-based perspective, one that recognizes individual agency and the role individuals must play in understanding, modifying, and adopting coping strategies and problem-solving skills that will foster positive change (Harris and Fallot 2001). This approach has also been defined as consisting of a "framework that is grounded in an understanding of and responsiveness to the impact of trauma, that emphasizes physical, psychological and emotional safety for both providers and survivors and that creates opportunities for survivors to rebuild a sense of control and empowerment" (Hopper, Bassuk, and Olivet 2010, p. 82). Rather than treating distress as a symptom of a disease, or problematic behaviors as signs of personal pathology, a program of trauma-informed care treats cognitive, emotional, interpersonal, and other difficulties as responses to managing victimization, social marginalization, economic disenfranchisement, and other forms of adversity that homeless citizens face (Hopper, Bassuk, and Olivet 2010; McManus and Thompson 2008). This approach also entails an emphasis on empowerment (as evinced in the case of several of the women, such as Debra and Freda, who are actively involved in therapeutic processes), including maximizing individual choice and autonomy, the removal of hierarchical boundaries between service providers and clients, active collaboration, and, of course, mutual commitment to healing (McManus and Thompson 2008).

Beyond these key organizing principles, trauma-informed care is often coupled with dialectical or cognitive behavioral forms of therapy, each of which aims to equip individuals with the skills they need to manage and ultimately overcome trauma and adversity. Both cognitive behavioral therapy and dialectical behavioral therapy have been subjected to control group research; the results of these studies lend support to the contention that these modes of therapy can succeed in helping traumatized individuals overcome a wide array of symptoms associated with traumatic distress. Such symptoms include, but are not limited to, suicidal ideation, self-harming behaviors, drug use, and eating disorders, among others (Black et al. 2012; Gosch et al. 2006; Harned et al. 2010; Landes and Linehan 2012).

Stable housing also has a crucial role to play in helping traumatized, impoverished women to recover and grow. As the women in this study revealed in Chapter 3, life on the streets and in shelters is fraught with tensions that create chronic stress for the individual, tensions that range from interpersonal conflicts with other shelter residents to random violence on the streets. Lack of privacy and autonomy also contribute to stress. So too do shelter policies that return women to the streets after they have exceeded the time limits on their stay and exhausted all other avenues of assistance. Throw in the fact that many of these same individuals have slept rough, and thus been exposed to the elements or to potential or real victimization on the streets, and one can easily see why mental well-being would be impaired as a result of being unhoused or temporarily housed within a shelter. Stable housing also contributes to physical health. Many of the women in this study were dealing with diabetes, hypertension, cancer, and other chronic health conditions, yet existing in spaces where they were without adequate rest and nutrition.[5] Perhaps the best illustration of the detrimental health impacts of homelessness are the lists, discussed in Chapter 5, that some of the women interviewed carried in order to follow the prescription regimens for the plethora of psychiatric and nonpsychiatric drugs they are taking. Having a secure home is one step in this direction; working to find avenues through which impoverished women can access healthy, quality foods is another.[6]

For anyone who recognizes that adverse living conditions can result in depression and anxiety and exacerbate symptoms associated with other mental health conditions, removing women from insecure, stressful living situations obviously must be a key ingredient of any attempt to address homelessness and the conditions that underpin this state. We are hardly alone in highlighting the importance of providing stable housing to individuals with complex needs. An entire body of literature demonstrates not only the personal and social benefits of housing provision to marginalized populations but also the importance of the timing of housing-based interventions (Appel et al. 2012; Collins, Malone, and Clifasefi 2013; Montgomery et al. 2013; Padgett, Gulcur, and Tsemberis 2006; Palepu et al. 2013; Patterson et al. 2013; Tsai, Mares, and Rosenheck 2010). Proponents of housing first are of the view that the traditional treatment-first orientation of many housing programs, which entails living in a shelter until one is judged stable, does not work in many instances and only contributes to the significant volume of individuals who cycle in and out of homelessness. By way of contrast, housing-first programs have shown the effectiveness, as measured principally by housing retention rates, client quality-of-life surveys, and rates of treatment compliance, of placing people into housing first and then attending to their other issues (Appel et al. 2012; Patterson et al. 2013; Tsemberis, Gulcur, and Nakae 2004). Given the seeming ineffectiveness of alternate models that prioritize so-called client stability over housing, we can only be in favor of approaches that remove traumatized individuals from situations that are known to create or exacerbate emotional and mental stress and suffering, as is the case with those sleeping in the streets and in most shelters.

Although many women will benefit from the provision of stable housing alone, one must keep in mind that others, particularly those with more complex psychosocial needs, will require housing that is not only safe and stable but also tied to supportive care. The reality is that many women coping with the effects of untreated trauma repeatedly cycle in and out of housing situations and thus require individualized comprehensive support in order to boost their chances of successfully turning the corner on the problems with which they grapple. In this situation, trauma-informed housing programs can be of critical assistance by "recognizing how the after-effects of trauma have contributed to residential instability, reframing these problematic behaviors as coping strategies, and promoting the development and application of new self-management skills in the housing environment" (Bebout 2001, p. 47). In essence, "house settings that are genuinely trauma informed offer trauma survivors the opportunity to acquire and practice new self-management and relationship skills and to experience 'home' in new ways" (Bebout 2001, p. 55).

A growing body of research also demonstrates that a significant component of fostering resiliency in individuals—that is, the ability to move beyond trauma and, in some cases, into posttraumatic growth—is contingent on access to positive supports within social networks and local communities (Joseph 2011; Ungar 2013). For this reason, it does not seem coincidental that the women in this study, such as Debra, who have developed new networks of friends and social activities from which they derive both personal support and positive feedback feel they are overcoming the lingering effects of abuse and other traumas. Nor is it accidental that women like Kathy are experiencing both improved mood and enhanced self-esteem through participation in fun and creative solo and group activities, as these activities provide both an opportunity for interacting positively with others and for expressing oneself in a safe space. In both instances, these new people and activities have replaced maladaptive coping strategies, including drugs and alcohol, as well as dysfunctional interpersonal relationships. Any serious attempt at addressing the roots of trauma among homeless citizens must therefore be based on an awareness of the need for comprehensive social supports within communities and for programs that build and nurture positive social connections between individuals and between individuals and groups.

As such, in the future, we encourage researchers to examine homelessness across different cities and subpopulations of women, including those with and without supports, to run comparison studies between the homeless women using psychiatric drugs and those who are not and to include long-term follow-ups (i.e., longitudinal studies) to see the trajectory of women in both subgroups. We suggest researchers study when and how different therapies and approaches to counseling can be most effective in treating women in need or with histories of trauma as well as study the effectiveness and best uses of diverse drugs for such populations. Further, we suggest researchers look to garner more insight into who is responsible for prescribing such medications in isolation (without therapy) and the rationale behind such practices to determine if the use of such medications is just a way to treat patients or perhaps another way in which structural violence is exhibited in societies.

Overall, we recognize the role for prescribed psychiatric drugs, particularly as a temporary response to an immediate state of crisis, or, in other words, when sedation is clearly called for in order to immediately lessen significant mental and emotional suffering or to prevent the individual from harming herself or others. However, as a long-term strategy for responding to the complex needs of homeless citizens, the resort to biopsychiatry and the use of psychiatric drugs in isolation is a public policy failure and yet another example of society's inability or unwillingness to invest in meaningful social change.

Notes

1. Medicalization runs rampant and includes normal conditions such as menopause, normal pregnancy, infertility, ADHD, erectile dysfunction, anxiety and behavioral disorders, body image, male pattern baldness, normal sadness, sleep disorders, and substance abuse disorders (Conrad and Barker 2010; Conrad, Mackie, and Mehrotra 2010).

2. We should point out that we are hardly antiscience. Indeed, when boarding a plane, we do so with a certain level of faith in the science of aerodynamics, including a belief that it is based on a fairly stable foundation of empirical observation and testing. However, we are not fans of blind trust, and therefore our faith in the laws of aerodynamics will not prevent us from looking over the weather forecast.

3. Canadians are routinely treated to an ad for a website called DepressionHurts.ca, which tells them that if a person *thinks* he or she might be suffering from the effects of depression, that person is not alone and can get helpful advice on treating the (as yet undiagnosed) depression. The website, which as of January 2014 had over 1 million visitors, entreats the readers to go "and talk to their doctor." As is the case with the television commercial, to which the viewers have been repeatedly and involuntarily subjected, the website contains no open identification of its owner. After wading through material on "the science behind depression" and "finding the right medication," a reader will discover the answer under the copyright section: the site is owned by an unnamed pharmaceutical company.

4. One of the shelters within which this study was conducted ran one of the largest and best-run psychological counseling programs in Los Angeles County. Staffed by a clinical director, a psychologist, counseling interns, and social workers, it provided trauma-informed therapy to clients in both individual counseling and group therapy sessions. Even some of the most therapy-resistant of their clients expressed respect for "Ms. T" and "Dr. K," who ran the program, and were even willing to confide in them things they might not have otherwise shared. Over the course of several months, the program was effectively gutted as a result of critical staff departures and absences.

Although we could not get the full story on what happened, two sources intimated that budget issues had forced cuts.

5. Recent scholarship on chronically homeless citizens has found that such individuals constitute a small proportion of the homeless population yet are responsible for a disproportionate amount of service use (see Kuhn and Culhane 1998). It also reveals that those who are "structurally homeless" (i.e., have lost their job, cannot afford housing, or have been cut off from welfare) will not qualify for housing-first programs in some places (Tsemberis, Gulcur, and Nakae 2004).

6. Having seen and tasted the food served at some places, one can easily state that it is typically not made from farm-fresh, quality ingredients, nor is it cooked in the most nutritional manner (being loaded with empty carbs, salt, and trans fats). Indeed, one day the lunch at a shelter we were working in was hot dogs. Several of the residents at this place told research team members they were sometimes left hungry because of a lack of food, and we noted that, had they the funds, the nearest eatery within walking distance was McDonald's, which was not an improvement.

Appendix: Research Methods

Collection of the data for the study that informs this book took place between August 2013 and August 2014. A research team consisting of one of the authors and five graduate student researchers made three separate visits to Los Angeles to conduct in-depth qualitative interviews with 201 ($n = 201$) women who used the services of either homeless shelters or transitional housing in the Los Angeles County.[1]

As was stated in Chapter 1, the purpose of the original study was to explore trauma and resiliency, with a particular focus on coping strategies. To that end, women interviewed for this study spoke of their experiences of various forms of trauma, most notably of victimization in both childhood and adulthood (intimate partner violence, sexual abuse, physical assault, sexual assault, or witnessing significant violence). They also discussed at length the various forms of coping they employed to deal with or to overcome the effects of trauma. Beyond the various personal coping strategies women adopted, one of the most frequently cited coping mechanisms was the use of psychiatric drugs.

Data Collection

To locate potential research participants, a nonprobability sample was developed that consisted of the maximum number of shelters and transitional housing programs for homeless women in Los Angeles (facilities that house either only women or both genders). These organizations were approached to see if they would agree to participate in the study by facilitating access to their clients. In total, eight agencies agreed.

Once present on-site, the research team introduced themselves, stated the purposes of the project, and then waited for individuals to self-select for participation in an interview. Once a woman approached and agreed to participate, she was again briefed on the study and its purposes. Criteria for inclusion included that each participant was a minimum age of eighteen years old, using the services of the selected agency, and appeared to be capable of providing informed consent.[2] All women who spoke to an interviewer were provided with a choice of a $10 gift card for either McDonald's or Walgreens.[3]

On average, interviews were typically forty minutes in duration and were conducted using an interview guide. Each team member received pre-field training in qualitative interviewing techniques and received further training and supervision in the field on technique and use of the interview guide under the guidance of two experienced team members. The interview guide consisted of questions related to the following areas: (1) demographic information, (2) traumatic events over the life course, (3) participant self-identification as "strong," "weak," or "in between" (resilient or not resilient), (4) resiliency determinants (personality characteristics), (5) resiliency processes (coping skills), and (6) suggestions for services. The bulk of the material presented in this book is drawn from answers provided to questions on experiences of trauma over the life course, coping strategies, and suggestions for services. All interviews were audio recorded with participants' consent and subsequently transcribed.

Data Analysis

To code and analyze the data collected, thematic analysis was employed (Braun and Clarke 2006). In the first stages of coding, an inductive approach was used. First, participant responses, as indicated by an interviewer on the interview guide, were coded. This first coding step resulted in a data set that provided basic information regarding demographic factors (a woman's age, length of current homelessness), types of trauma experienced, coping skills used, and so on. These results were subsequently verified against transcripts of the interviews.

To develop a set of thematic codes from the interviews, we relied on two sources: notes taken during postinterview team debriefing sessions (during which team members discussed their impressions of an interview and what they saw as interesting or salient points from that interview), and notes taken during initial readings of transcripts. In relation to coping strategies, psychiatric drug use was repeatedly identified in both sources and thus became a major theme in our analysis. Once initial coding was complete, we evaluated our preliminary results and began the process of developing a suitable theoretical framework to help deepen our understanding of what the data was revealing about the use of psychiatric drugs for the treatment of trauma within this population. Further focused coding allowed us to refine our ideas and to assess the extent to which our data fit with the framework employed as well as the existing research literature.

Notes

1. This study was subject to institutional ethics review and was conducted in accordance with Canadian Tri-Council research ethics guidelines.

2. The last was determined by whether a woman appeared sober and lucid during the preinterview discussion. If she did not appear capable of giving informed consent during the preinterview, she was thanked for her time and presented with a $10 gift card.

3. The amount of the gift card was determined based on funds available and the research project costs (e.g., research assistant wages and transcription and travel costs), which were not insignificant.

References

Abdul-Hamid, W., and Bhui, K. 2014. "Psychiatry, Homeless Patients and Welfare Reforms: Historical Links and Chains." *International Journal of Social Psychiatry* 60(1): 71–74.

Ahn, W., Proctor, C., and Flanagan, E. 2009. "'Mental Health Clinicians' Beliefs About the Biological, Psychological, and Environmental Bases of Mental Disorders." *Cognitive Science* 33(2): 147–182.

Aho, K. 2008. "Medicalizing Mental health: A Phenomenological Alternative." *Journal of Medical Humanities* 29(4): 243–259.

Albee, G., and Joffe, J. 2004. "Mental Illness Is NOT 'an Illness Like Any Other.'" *Journal of Primary Prevention* 24(4): 419–436.

Amato, F., and Macdonald, J. 2011. "Examining Risk Factors for Homeless Men: Gender Role Conflict, Help-Seeking Behaviors, Substance Abuse and Violence." *Journal of Men's Studies* 19(3): 227–235.

Ambrosio, E., Baker, D., Crowe, C., and Hardill, K. 1992. *The Street Health Report: A Study of the Health Status and Barriers to Health Care of Homeless Women and Men in the City of Toronto*. Toronto, ON: Street Health.

Andreasen, N. C., Carpenter Jr, W. T., Kane, J. M., Lasser, R. A., Marder, S. R., and Weinberger, D. R. 2005. "Remission in Schizophrenia: Proposed Criteria and Rationale for Consensus." *American Journal of Psychiatry* 162(3): 441–449.

Andrews, G., Issakidis, C., and Carter, G. 2001. "Shortfall in Mental Health Service Utilisation." *British Journal of Psychiatry* 179: 417–425.

Angell, M. 2000. "Is Academic Medicine for Sale?" *New England Journal of Medicine* 342: 1516–1519.

APA (American Psychiatric Association). 2010. "Detail on Industry Revenue 2010." http://www.psychiatry.org.

———. 2012. "Detail on Industry Revenue 2012." http://www.psychiatry.org.

———. 2013. *Diagnostic and Statistical Manual of Mental Disorders*, 5th ed. Washington, DC: APA.

———. 2015. "History of the Diagnostic and Statistical Manual on Mental Illness." http://www.psychiatry.org.

Appel, P., Tsemberis, S., Joseph, H., Stefancic, A., and Lambert-Wacey, D. 2012. "Housing First for Severely Mentally Ill Homeless Methadone Patients." *Journal of Addictive Diseases* 31(3): 270–277.

Appelbaum, P. 2003. "Ambivalence Codified: California's New Outpatient Commitment Statute." *Psychiatric Services* 54(1): 26–28.

Armstrong, P., and Armstrong, H. 2010. *Wasting Away: The Undermining of Canadian Health Care*. Wynford Project Edition. Toronto, ON: Oxford University Press.

Arroyo, J. 1996. "Psychotherapist Bias with Hispanics: An Analog Study." *Hispanic Journal of Behavioural Sciences* 18(1): 21–28.

Austin, E., Andersen, R., and Gelberg, L. 2008. "Ethnic Differences in the Correlates of Mental Distress Among Homeless Women." *Women's Health Issues* 18: 26–34.

Baer, H., Singer, M., and Susser, I. 1997. *Medical Anthropology and the World System*. Westport, CT: Greenwood.

Ban, T. 2007. "Fifty Years of Chlorpromazine: A Historical Perspective." *Neuropsychiatric Disease and Treatment* 3(4): 495–500.

Barber, C. 2009. *Comfortably Numb: How Psychiatry Is Medicating a Nation*. New York: Pantheon.

Barrow, S., and Laborde, N. 2008. "Invisible Mothers: Parenting by Homeless Women Separated from Their Children." *Gender Issues* 25: 157–172.

Bassuk, E., Buckner, J., Perloff, J., and Bassuk, S. 1998. "Prevalence of Mental Health and Substance Use Disorders Among Homeless and Low-Income Housed Mothers." *American Journal of Psychiatry* 155(11): 1561–1564.

Bayer, R., and Spitzer, R. 1985. "Neurosis, Psychodynamics, and DSM-III: A History of the Controversy." *Archives of General Psychiatry* 42(2): 187–196.

Bebout, R. 2001. "Trauma-Informed Approaches." *New Directions in Mental Health Services* 89: 47–55.

Becker, D., and Lamb, S. 1994. "Sex Bias in the Diagnosis of Borderline Personality Disorder and Post-Traumatic Stress Disorder." *Professional Psychology: Research and Practice* 25(1): 55–61.

Bell, C., Williamson, J., and Chien, P. 2008. "Cultural, Racial and Ethnic Competence and Psychiatric Diagnosis." *Ethnicity and Inequalities in Health and Social Care* 1(1): 34–41.

Ben-Moshe, L., Chapman, C., and Carey, A. C., Eds. 2014. *Disability Incarcerated: Imprisonment and Disability in the United States and Canada*. New York: Palgrave Macmillan.

Bentall, R. P. 2009. *Doctoring the Mind: Why Psychiatric Treatments Fail*. London: Penguin.

Bjorklund, P. 2005. "'Can There be a 'Cosmetic' Psychopharmacology? Prozac Unplugged: The Search for an Ontologically Distinct Cosmetic Psychopharmacology.'" *Nursing Philosophy* 6: 131–143.

Black, P., Woodworth, M. Tremblay, M., and Carpenter, T. 2012. "A Review of Trauma-Informed Treatment for Adolescents." *Canadian Psychology* 53(3): 192–203.

Bloom, S. L. 2009. "An Elephant In The Room: The Impact Of Traumatic Stress On Individuals and Groups," in K. Brown and B. Bergo, eds., *The Trauma Controversy: Philosophical and Interdisciplinary Dialogues*, 143–169. Albany: SUNY Press.

Bourgois, P. 1998. "Ethnography of Substance Use: The Moral Economies of Homeless Heroin Addicts: Confronting Ethnography, HIV Risk, and Everyday Violence in San Francisco Shooting Encampments." *Substance Use and Misuse* 33(1): 2323–2351.

Bourgois, P., Prince, B., and Moss, A. 2004. "The Everyday Violence of Hepatitis C Among Young Women Who Inject Drugs in San Francisco." *Human Organization* 63(3): 253–262.

Bowden, G. 2014. "The Merit of Sociological Account of Disorder: The Attention-Deficit Hyperactivity Disorder Case." *Health* (London) 18(4): 422–438.

Braun, V., and Clarke, V. 2006. "Using Thematic Analysis in Psychology." *Qualitative Research in Psychology* 3(2): 77–101.

Breggin, P. 1991. *Toxic Psychiatry*. New York: St. Martin's.

Breslau, N., Chilcocat, H., Kessler, R., and Davis, G. 1999. "Previous Exposure to Trauma and PTSD Effects of Subsequent Trauma: Results from the Detroit Area Survey of Trauma." *American Journal of Psychiatry* 156: 902–907.

Bresnahan, M., Begg, M., Brown, A., Schaefer, C., Sohler, N., Insel, B., Vella, L., and Susser, E. 2007. "Race and Risk of Schizophrenia in a US Birth Cohort: Another Example of Health Disparity?" *International Journal of Epidemiology* 36(40): 751–758.

Brewerton, T. D. 1994. "Hyperreligiosity in Psychotic Disorder." *Journal of Nervous and Mental Disease* 182(5): 302–304.

Brodwin, P. 2010. "The Assemblage of Compliance in Psychiatric Case Management." *Anthropology and Medicine* 17(2): 129–143.

Brown, P. 1993. "Psychiatric Intake as a Mystery Story." *Culture, Medicine and Psychiatry* 17: 255–280.

Browne, A., and Bassuk, S. 1997. "Intimate Violence in the Lives of Homeless and Poor Housed Women: Prevalence and Patterns in an Ethnically Diverse Sample." *American Journal of Orthopsychiatry* 67(2): 261–278.

Browne, C., and Winkelman, C. 2007. "The Effect of Childhood Trauma on Later Psychological Adjustment." *Journal of Interpersonal Violence* 22(6): 684–697.

Bullock, H. 2004. "Diagnosis of Low-Income Women," in P. Caplan and L. Cosgrove, eds., *Bias in Psychiatric Diagnosis*, 115–120. Oxford: Rowman and Littlefield.

Campbell, L. 2010, February 26. "Paxil Suicide Lawsuit Can Go Ahead." *Lawyers andSettlements.com*. http://www.lawyersandsettlements.com/articles/paxil_suicide/Paxil-suicide-lawsuit-13678.html#.VPR7EPnF-So (accessed September 13, 2015).

Canto, V. A., Jones, D. H., and Laffer, A. B. 1983. *Foundations of Supply-Side Economics*. New York: Academic.

Cardno, A., Sham, P., Gottesman, I., Framer, A., and McGuffin, P. 1999. "Heritability Estimates for Psychotic Disorders: The Maudsley Twin Psychosis Series." *Archives of General Psychiatry* 56(2): 162–168.

Chesler, P. 2005 [1972]. *Women and Madness*. New York: Palgrave Macmillan.

Choong, E., Bondol, G., Etter, M., Jermann, F., Aubry, J., Bartolomei, J., Gholam-Rezaee, M., and Eap, C. 2012. "Psychotropic Drug-Induced Weight Gain and Other Metabolic Complications in a Swiss Psychiatric Population." *Journal of Psychiatric Research* 46: 540–548.

Chrisler, J., and Caplan, P. 2002. "The Strange Case of Dr. Jekyll and Ms. Hyde: How PMS Became a Cultural Phenomenon and a Psychiatric Disorder." *Annual Review of Sex Research* 13: 274–306.

Chung, J. Y., Frank, L., Subramanian, A., Galen, S., Leonhard, S., and Green B. L. 2012. "A Qualitative Evaluation of Barriers to Care for Truma-Related Mental Health Problems Among Low-Income Minorities in Primary Care." *Journal of Nervous and Mental Disease* 200(5): 438–443.

Cloke, P., May, J., and Johnsen, S. 2010. *Swept Up Lives? Re-Envisioning the Homeless City*. Chichester, UK: Wiley Blackwell.

Collins, S., Malone, D., and Clifasefi, S. 2013. "Housing Retention in Single-Site Housing First for Chronically Homeless Individuals with Severe Alcohol Problems." *American Journal of Public Health* 103(2): S269–S274.

———. 2010, May 18. "Peter Conrad Studies the Medicalization of Human Problems." *Brandeis Now*. http://www.brandeis.edu/now/2010/may/medicalizationrelease .html (accessed September 13, 2015).

Conrad, P., and Barker, K. K. 2010. "The Social Construction of Illness: Key Insights and Policy Implications." *Journal of Health and Social Behavior* 51(1): 567–579.

Conrad, P., Mackie, T., and Mehrotra, A. 2010. "Estimating the Costs of Medicalization." *Social Science and Medicine* 70(12): 1943–1947.

Conrad, P., and Schneider, J. 1992. *Deviance and Medicalization: From Badness to Sickness*. Philadelphia: Temple University Press.

Correll, C., and Schenk, E. 2008. "Tardive Dyskinesia and New Antipsychotics." *Current Opinion in Psychiatry* 21(2): 151–156.

Dalky, H. F. 2012. "Mental Illness Stigma Reduction Interventions: Review of Intervention Trials." *Western Journal of Nursing Research* 34(4): 520–547.

Davies-Netzley, S., Hurlburt, M., and Hough, R. 1996. "Childhood Abuse as a Precursor to Homelessness for Homeless Women with Severe Mental Illness." *Violence and Victims* 11(2): 129–142.

Davis, V., and Rosenbloom, A. 2006. "Metabolic Effects of Antipsychotic Drugs." *Pediatric Diabetes* 7: 176–186.

Dear, M., and Wolch, J. 1987. *Landscapes of Despair: From Deinstitutionalization to Homelessness*. Princeton: Princeton University Press.

D'Ercole, A., and Struening, E. 1990. "Victimization Among Homeless Women: Implications for Service Delivery." *Journal of Community Psychology* 18(2): 141–152.

Demler, T. L. 2014. "Drug-Induced Neurologic Conditions." *US Pharmacist* 39(1): 47–52.

DeVerteuil, G., and Wilton, R. 2009. "Spaces of Abeyance, Care and Survival: The Addiction Treatment System as a Rite of 'Regulatory Richness.'" *Political Geography* 28(8): 463–472.

Ditlevsen, D., and Elklit, A. 2010. "The Combined Effect of Gender and Age on Post Traumatic Stress Disorder: Do Men and Women Show Differences in the Lifespan Distribution of the Disorder?" *Annals of General Psychiatry* 9(1): 32–44.

Dixon, L., Friedman, N., and Lehman, A. 1993. "Compliance of Homeless Mentally Ill Persons with Assertive Community Treatment." *Psychiatric Services* 44(6): 581–583.

Dixon, L., Weiden, P., Torres, M., and Lehman, A. 1997. "Assertive Community Treatment and Medication Compliance in the Homeless Mentally Ill." *American Journal of Psychiatry* 154(9): 1302–1304.

Double, D. 2011. "Why Were Doctors So Slow to Recognize Antidepressant Discontinuation Problems?, in M. Rapley, J. Moncrieff, and J. Dillon, *De-Medicalizing Misery: Psychiatry, Psychology and the Human Condition*, 197–210. London: Palgrave Macmillan.

Eack, S., Bahorik, A., Newhill, C., Neighbors, H., and Davis, L. 2012. "Interviewer-Perceived Honesty as a Mediator of Racial Disparities in the Diagnosis of Schizophrenia." *Psychiatric Services* 63(9): 875–880.

Ehrenreich, D., and English, D. 2005. *For Her Own Good: Centuries of the Experts' Advice to Women*. New York: Anchor.

Elzy, M., Clark, C., Dollard, N., and Hummer, V. 2013. "Adolescent Girls' Use of Avoidant and Approach Coping as Moderators Between Trauma Exposure and Trauma Symptoms." *Journal of Family Violence* 28: 763–770.

Esquivel, P. 2014, March 9. "Kelly Thomas Case Prompts Counties to Take Fresh Look at Laura's Law." *LA Times*. http://articles.latimes.com/2014/mar/09/local/la-me-adv-lauras-law-20140310 (accessed December 14, 2015).

Etain, B., Aas, M., Andreassen, O. A., Lorentzen, S., Dieset, I., Gard, S., Kahn, J. P., Bellivier, F., Leboyer, M., Melle, I., Henry, C. 2013. "Childhood Trauma Is Associated with Severe Clinical Characteristics of Bipolar Disorders." *Journal of Clinical Psychiatry* 74(10): 991–998.

Etain, B., Henry, C., Bellivier, F., Mathieu, F., and Leboyer, M. 2008. "Beyond Genetics: Childhood Affective Trauma in Bipolar Disorder." *Bipolar Disorders* 10(8): 867–876.

Fairbanks, R. P. 2009. *How It Works: Recovering Citizens in Post-Welfare Philadelphia*. Chicago: University of Chicago Press.

Farmer, P. 2004. "An Anthropology of Structural Violence." *Current Anthropology* 45(3): 205–324.

———. 2009. "On Suffering and Structural Violence: A View from Below." *Race and the Global Politics of Health* 3(1): 11–28.

Finfgeld-Connett, D. 2010. "Becoming Homeless, Being Homeless, and Resolving Homelessness Among Women." *Issues in Mental Health Nursing* 31(7): 461–469.

Ford, M., and Widiger, T. 1989. "Sex Bias in the Diagnosis of Histrionic and Antisocial Personality Disorders." *Journal of Consulting and Clinical Psychology* 57(2): 301–305.

France, C. M., Lysaker, P. H., and Robinson, Ryan P. 2007. "The 'Chemical Imbalance' Explanation for Depression: Origins, Lay Endorsement, and Clinical Implications. *Professional Psychology: Research and Practice* 38(4): 411–420.

Frances, A. 2013. *Saving Normal*. New York: William Morrow.

Freeman, D., and Fowler, D. 2009. "Routes to Psychotic Symptoms: Trauma, Anxiety, and Psychosis-Like Experiences." *Psychiatry Residents* 169(2): 107–112.

Freemantle, N., and Mason, J. 2000. "The Importance of Achieving Additional Drug Benefits at a Reasonable Cost: A Review of the Fluoxetine Years." *Pharmacoeconomics* 17(4): 319–324.

Freyd, J. 1994. "Betrayal Trauma: Traumatic Amnesia as an Adaptive Response to Childhood Abuse." *Ethics and Behavior* 4(4): 307–329.

Fried, J., Harris, B., Evles, J., and Moshabela, M. 2015. "Acceptable Care? Illness Constructions, Health Worlds, and Accessible Chronic Treatment in South Africa." *Qualitative Health Research* 25(5): 622–635.
Friedman, R. A. 2014. "Antidepressants' Black-Box Warning—10 Years Later." *New England Journal of Medicine* 371: 1666–1668.
Fujioka, W. 2012, March 20. "Memorandum: Sacramento Update." http://file.lacounty.gov/bc/q1_2012/cms1_176157.pdf (accessed September 13, 2015).
Fuller Torrey, E. 1988. *Nowhere to Go: The Tragic Odyssey of the Homeless Mentally Ill*. New York: Harper and Row.
———. 2006. *Surviving Schizophrenia*, 5th ed. New York: HarperCollins.
Gardos, G. 1999. "Managing Antipsychotic-Induced Tardive Dyskinesia." *Drug Safety* 20(2): 187–193.
Gershon, A., Johnson, S. L., and Miller, I. 2013. "Chronic Stressors and Trauma: Prospective Influences on the Course of Bipolar Disorder." *Psychology of Medicine* 43(12): 2583–9252.
Ghafoori, B., Barragan, B., and Palinkas, L. 2013. "Gender Disparities in the Mental Health of Urban Survivors of Trauma." *Journal of Aggression, Maltreatment and Trauma* 22: 950–963.
Giordano, J., Ed. 2012. *Advances in Neurotechnology: Premises, Potential and Problems*. Boca Raton, FL: CRC.
Goffman, E. 1963. *Stigma: Notes on the Management of the Spoiled Identity*. New York: Prentice Hall.
Gold, S. D., Marx B. P., Soler-Baillo, J. M., Sloan, D. M. 2005. "Is Life Stress More Traumatic Than Traumatic Stress." *Journal of Anxiety Disorders* 19(6): 687–698.
Gosch, E., Flannery-Shroeder, E., Maura, C., and Compton, S. 2006. "Principles of Cognitive-Behavioral Therapy for Anxiety Disorders in Children." *Journal of Cognitive Psychotherapy* 20: 247–262.
Gowan, T. 2010. *Hobos, Hustlers, and Backsliders: Homelessness in San Francisco*. Minneapolis: University of Minnesota Press.
Greenberg, G. 2013. *The Book of Woe: The DSM and the Unmaking of Psychiatry*. New York: Blue Rider.
Greifenhagen, A., and Fichter, M. 1997. "Mental Illness in Homeless Women: An Epidemiological Study in Munich, Germany." *European Archives of Psychiatry and Clinical Neuroscience* 247(3): 162–172.
Gu, Q., Dillon, C., and Burt, V. 2010. "Prescription Drug Use Continues to Increase: U.S. Prescription Drug Data for 2007–2008." *NCHS Data Brief*, 42. http://www.cdc.gov/nchs/data/databriefs/db42.html (accessed November 20, 2013).
Gueorguieva, R., Mallinckrodt, C., and Krystal, J. 2011. "Trajectories of Depression Severity in Clinical Trials of Duloxetine: Insights into Antidepressant and Placebo Responses." *Archives of General Psychiatry* 68(12): 1227–1237.
Gupta, A. 2013. "Structural Violence and Politics." *Economy and Society* 42(4): 686–692.
Hacking, I. 1995. *Rewriting the Soul*. Princeton: Princeton University Press.
Haddad, P. M., and Dursun, S. M. 2008. "Neurological Complications of Psychiatric Drugs: Clinical Features and Management." *Human Psychopharmacology* 23(1): 15–26.

Hammersket, P., Dias, A., Todd, G., et al. (2003). "Childhood Trauma and Hallucinations in Bipolar Affective Disorder: Preliminary Investigation." *British Journal of Psychiatry* 182: 543–547.

Hammersley, P., Dias, A., Todd, G., Bowen-Jones, K., Reilly, B., Bentall, R. P. 2003. "Childhood Trauma and Hallucinations in Bipolar Affective Disorder: Preliminary Investigation." *British Journal of Psychiatry* 182: 543–547.

Harned, M., Jackson, S., Comtois, K., and Linehan, M. 2010. "Dialectical Behavior Therapy as a Precursor to PTSD Treatment for Suicidal and/or Self-Injuring Women with Borderline Personality Disorder." *Journal of Traumatic Stress* 23(4): 421–442.

Harris, M., and Fallot, R. 2001. *Using Trauma Theory to Design Service Systems.* San Francisco: Jossey-Bass.

Hausken, A., Furu, K., Tverdal, A., and Skurtveit, S. 2010. "Mental Distress and Subsequent Use of Anxiolytic Drugs—A Prospective Population-Based Cohort Study of 16,000 Individuals." *Scandinavian Journal of Public Health* 38: 465–473.

Hausken A., Skurtveit S., and Tverdal, A. 2007. "Use of Anxiolytic or Hypnotic Drugs and Total Mortality in a General Middle-Aged Population." *Pharmacoepidemiological Drug Safety* 16(8): 913–918.

Healy, D. 2004. *Let Them Eat Prozac: The Unhealthy Relationship Between the Pharmaceutical Industry and Depression.* New York: New York University Press.

———. 2012. *Pharmageddon.* Oakland: University of California Press.

Heitt, S., Graham, Y., and Nemeroff, C. B. 1999. "Neurobiological Effects of Early Trauma." *The Harvard Mental Health Letter, from Harvard Medical School* 16(4): 4–6.

———. 2013. *Pharmageddon.* Berkeley: University of California Press.

Herman, J. 1992. *Trauma and Recovery: The Aftermath of Violence—Domestic Abuse to Political Terror.* New York: Basic Books.

Herrenkohl, T., Sousa, C., Tajima, E., Herrenkohl, R., and Moylan, C. 2008. "Intersection of Child Abuse and Children's Exposure to Domestic Violence." *Trauma, Violence, and Abuse* 9(2): 84–99.

Hesslow, G. 1993. "Do We Need a Concept of Disease?" *Theoretical Medicine* 14: 1–14.

Hetzel-Riggin, M., and Roby, R. 2013. "Trauma Type and Gender Effects on PTSD, General Distress, and Peritraumatic Dissociation." *Journal of Loss and Trauma* 18(1): 41–53.

Hitchens, C. 2012. *Mortality.* New York: Twelve.

Hodgetts, D., Chamberlain, K., Groot, S., and Tankel, Y. 2014. "Urban Poverty, Structural Violence and Welfare Provisions for 100 Families in Auckland." *Urban Studies* 51(10): 2036–2051.

Holt, R., and Peveler, R. 2011. "Antipsychotics and Hyperprolactinaemia: Mechanisms, Consequences and Management." *Clinical Endocrinology* 74(2): 141–147.

Hopper, E., Bassuk, E., and Olivet, J. 2010. "Shelter from the Storm: Trauma-Informed Care in Homelessness Services." *Open Health Services and Policy Journal* 3(1): 80–100.

Hudson, A., Wright, K., Battacharya, D., Sinha, K., Nyamathi, A., and Marfisee, M. 2010. "Correlates of Adult Assault Among Homeless Women." *Journal of Health Care for the Poor and Underserved* 21(4): 1250–1262.

Huey, L., Fthenos, G., and Hryniewicz, D. 2012. "'I Need Help and I Know I Need Help. Why Won't Nobody Listen to Me?': Homeless Women's Experiences with Accessing and Consuming Mental Health Services." *Society and Mental Health* 2(2): 120–134.

———. 2013. "'If Something Happened, I Will Leave It, Let It Go and Move On': Resiliency and Victimized Homeless Women's Attitudes Toward Mental Health Counseling." *Journal of Interpersonal Violence* 28(2): 294–318.

Hughes, A., Lynch, P., and Yates, R. 1999. "Electroencephalographic and Psychomotor Effects of Chlorpromazine and Risperidone Relative to Placebo in Normal Healthy Volunteers." *British Journal of Clinical Pharmacology* 48(3): 323–330.

Hughes, S., and Peak, T. 2013. "A Critical Perspective on the Role of Psychotropic Medications in Mental Health Courts." *American Behavioral Scientist* 57(2): 244–265.

IMS Institute for Healthcare Informatics. 2014. "The Use of Medicines in the United States: Review of 2013." http://www.imshealth.com/deployedfiles/imshealth/Global/Content/Corporate/IMS%20Health%20Institute/Reports/Secure/IIHI_US_Use_of_Meds_for_2013.pdf (accessed June 26, 2014).

Janoff-Bulman, R. 1992. *Shattered Assumptions: Towards a New Psychology of Trauma*. New York: Free Press.

Jarvis, W. T. 1996. "'Misuse of the Term 'Allopathy.'" http://www.ncahf.org/articles/a-b/allopathy.html (accessed September 13, 2015).

Jasinski, J., Wesely, J., Wright, J., and Mustaine, E. 2010. *Hard Lives, Mean Streets: Violence in the Lives of Homeless Women*. Hanover, MA: Northeastern University Press.

Jencks, C. 1994. *The Homeless*. Cambridge, MA: Harvard University Press.

Johansen, V., Wahl, A., Eilertsen, D., and Weisaeth, L. 2007. "Prevalence and Predictors of Post-Traumatic Stress Disorder (PTSD) in Physically Injured Victims of Non-Domestic Violence: A Longitudinal Study." *Social Psychiatry and Psychiatric Epidemiology* 42: 583–593.

Johnsen, S., and Fitzpatrick, S. 2010. "Revanchist Sanitisation or Coercive Care? The Use of Enforcement to Combat Begging, Street Drinking and Rough Sleeping in England." *Urban Studies* 47(8): 1703–1723.

Jones, L., Hughes, M., and Unterstaller, U. 2001. "Post-Traumatic Stress Disorder (PTSD) in Victims of Domestic Violence: A Review of the Research." *Trauma, Violence, and Abuse* 2(2): 99–119.

Joseph, S. 2011. *What Doesn't Kill Us: The New Psychology of Posttraumatic Growth*. New York: Basic.

Karon, B. P. 2007. "Trauma and Schizophrenia." *Journal of Psychological Trauma* 6(2/3): 127–144.

Kaufman M. 1988. "Homeopathy in America: The Rise and Fall and Persistence of a Medical Heresy," in N. Gervitz, ed., *Other Healers: Unorthodox Medicine in America*, 99–123. Baltimore: Johns Hopkins University Press.

Kawa, S, and Giordano, J. 2012. "A Brief Historicity of the *Diagnostic and Statistical Manual of Mental Disorders*: Issues and Implications for the Future of

Psychiatric Canon and Practice." *Philosophy, Ethics and Humanity in Medicine* 7(2).

Kelly, B. D. 2005. "Structural Violence and Schizophrenia." *Social Science and Medicine* 61: 721–730.

Kendler, K. 2013. "What Psychiatric Genetics Has Taught Us About the Nature of Psychiatric Illness and What Is Left to Learn." *Molecular Psychiatry* 18: 1058–1066.

Kim, J. Y., Millen, J. V., Irwin, A., and Greshman, J., Eds. 2000. *Dying for Growth: Global Inequality and the Health of the Poor*. Monroe, ME: Common Cause.

Kirsch, I. 2010. *The Emperor's New Drugs: Exploding the Antidepressant Myth*. New York: Basic.

Koegel, P., Burnam, M., and Farr, R. 1988. "The Prevalence of Specific Psychiatric Disorders Among Homeless Individuals in the Inner City of Los Angeles." *Archives of General Psychiatry* 12: 1085–1092.

Kondrat, D. C., and Early, T. C. 2011. "Battling in the Trenches: Case Managers' Ability to Combat the Effects of Mental Illness Stigma on Consumers' Perceived Quality of Life." *Community Mental Health Journal* 47(4): 390–398.

Koopmans, G., and Lamers, L. 2007. "Gender and Health Care Utilization: The Role of Mental Distress and Help-Seeking Propensity." *Social Science and Medicine* 64: 1216–1230.

Kramer, P. 1993. *Listening to Prozac: A Psychiatrist Explores Antidepressant Drugs and the Remaking of the Self*. New York: Penguin Books.

Kreig, R. G. 2001. "An Interdisciplinary Look at the Deinstitutionalization of the Mentally Ill." *Social Science Journal* 38.

Kuhn, R., and Culhane, D. P. 1998. "Applying Cluster Analysis to Test a Typology of Homelessness by Pattern of Shelter Utilization: Results from the Analysis of Administrative Data." *American Journal of Community Psychology* 26(2): 207–232.

Kutchins, H., and Kirk, S. 1997. *Making Us Crazy: DSM: The Psychiatric Bible and the Creation of Mental Disorders*. New York: Simon and Schuster.

LACDMH (Los Angeles County Department of Mental Health). 2016. *Wellness and Client-Run Centers Brochure*. http://file.lacounty.gov/dmh/cms1_159263.pdf (accessed May 8, 2016).

———. 2013. *Laura's Law Implementation Model Project*. http://file.lacounty.gov/dmh/cms1_204073.pdf (accessed June 8, 2014).

Lam, J., and Rosenheck, R. 1998. "The Effect of Victimization on Clinical Outcomes of Homeless Persons with Serious Mental Illness." *Psychiatric Services* 49(5): 678–683.

Lamb, H., and Talbott, J. 1986. "The Homeless Mentally Ill: The Perspective of the American Psychiatric Association." *JAMA* 256(4): 498–501.

Lamb, H. R., and Bachrach, L. L. 2001. "Some Perspectives on Deinstitutionalization." *Psychiatry Services* 52(8): 1039–1045.

Landes, S., and Linehan, M. 2012. "Dissemination and Implementation of Dialectical Behavior Therapy: An Intensive Training Model," in D. Barlow and R. McHugh, eds., *Dissemination and Implementation of Evidence-Based Psychological Interventions*, 187–208. New York: Oxford University Press.

Lane, C. 2006. "How Shyness Became an Illness: A Brief History of Social Phobia." *Common Knowledge* 12(3): 388–409.

Larney, E., Conroy, K., Mills, L., and Teesson, M. 2009. "Factors Associated with Violent Victimisation Among Homeless Adults in Sydney, Australia." *Australian and New Zealand Journal of Public Health* 33(4): 347–351.

Launer, J. 2014. "On Reflection: Do Diseases Really Exist?' *Postgraduate Medical Journal* 90: 425–426.

Leo, R., and Del Regno, P. 2001. "Social Security Claims of Psychiatric Disability: Elements of Case Adjudication and the Role of Primary Care Physicians." *Primary Care Companion of Journal of Clinical Psychiatry* 3(6): 255–262.

Lindsay, K., Sankis, L., and Widiger, T. 2000. "Gender Bias in Self-Report Personality Disorder Inventories." *Journal of Personality Disorders* 14(3): 218–232.

Llorente, M., and Urrutia, V. 2006. "Diabetes, Psychiatric Disorders, and the Metabolic Effects of Antipsychotic Medications." *Clinical Diabetes* 24(1): 18–24.

Lovell, A. 1992. "Classification and Its Risks: How Psychiatric Status Contributes to Homelessness Policy." *New England Journal of Public Policy* 8(1): 247–263.

Lutfey, K. 2013. "Evaluating Sources and Implications of Doctor Bias." *Medical Education* 47(8): 756–758.

Lyng, S. 1990. *Holistic Health and Biomedical Medicine: A Counter Analysis*. Albany, NY: SUNY Press.

Lyon-Callo, V. 2008. *Inequality, Poverty, and Neoliberal Governance: Activist Ethnography in the Homeless Sheltering Industry*. Toronto, ON: University of Toronto Press.

Lysaker, P. H., and LaRocco, V. A. 2008. "The Prevalence and Correlates of Trauma-Related Symptoms in Schizophrenia Spectrum Disorder." *Comprehensive Psychiatry* 49(4): 330–334.

Markowitz, F. E. 2006. "Psychiatric Hospital Capacity, Homelessness, and Crime and Arrest Rates." *Criminology* 44: 45–72.

———. 2011. "Dysfunctional Social Control of Mental Illness." *Social Science and Medicine* 72: 456–459.

Marshall, K., Georgievskava, Z., and Georgievsky, I. 2009. "Social Reactions to Valium and Prozac: A Cultural Lag Perspective of Drug Diffusion and Adoption." *Research in Social and Administrative Pharmacy* 5(1): 94–107.

Marx, M., and McCravey, H. 2012, November 7. "AB 109: A Journey to Integration: From Incarceration to Community—A Collaborative Approach." Ninth Statewide Conference paper. http://www.uclaisap.org/slides/psattc/cod/2012/Workshop%20Session%20B/Workshop%20B%20-%20Day%201%20AB%20109%20Ninth%20Statewide%20Conference%20Presentation%20-%20Marx%20and%20McCravey.pdf (accessed June 23, 2016).

Mauritz, M. W., Goossens, P. J. J., Draijer, N., and van Achterberg, T. 2013. "Prevalence of Interpersonal Trauma Exposure and Trauma-Related Disorders in Severe Mental Illness." *European Journal of Psychotraumatol* 4(10).

McKenzie-Mohr, S., Coates, J., and McLeod, H. 2012. "Responding to the Needs of Youth Who Are Homeless: Calling for Politicized Trauma-Informed Intervention." *Children and Youth Services Review* 34: 136–143.

McManus, H., and Thompson, S. 2008. "Trauma Among Unaccompanied Homeless Youth: The Integration of Street Culture into a Model of Intervention." *Journal of Aggression, Maltreatment and Trauma* 16(1): 92–109.

Medco. 2011. "America's State of Mind." A Report by Medco. http://apps.who.int/medicinedocs/documents/s19032en/s19032en.pdf.

Moncrieff, J. 2011. "The Myth of the Antidepressant," in M. Rapley, J. Moncrieff, and J. Dillon, eds., *De-Medicalizing Misery*, 174–188. London: Palgrave Macmillan.

———. 2013. *The Bitterest Pills: The Troubling Story of Antipsychotic Drugs*. New York: Palgrave Macmillan.

Montgomery, A., Hill, L., Kane, V., and Culhane, D. 2013. "Housing Chronically Homeless Veterans: Evaluating the Efficacy of a Housing First Approach to HUD VASH." *Journal of Community Psychology* 41(4): 505–514.

Moskowitz, A., Schafer, I., and Dorahy, M. J., Eds. 2009. *Psychosis, Trauma, and Dissociation: Emerging Perspectives on Severe Psychopathology.* West Sussex: John Wiley.

Mowlds, W., Shannon, C., McCusker, C. G., Meenagh, C., Robinson, D., Wilson, A., Mulholland, C. 2010. "Autobiographical Memory: Specificity, Depression, and Trauma in Bipolar Disorder." *British Journal of Clinical Psychology* 49: 217–233.

Muir-Cochrane, E., Fereday, J., Jureidini, J., Drummond, A., and Darbyshire, P. 2006. "Self-Management of Medication for Mental Health Problems by Homeless Young People." *International Journal of Mental Health Nursing* 15(2): 163–170.

National Institute of Mental Health. 2014. "Mental Health Medications." http://www.nimh.nih.gov/health/publications/mental-health-medications/index.shtml (accessed May 8, 2016).

Nicholas, B. 2009. "The Impact of Uncertainty Shocks." *Econometrica, Econometric Society* 77(3): 623–685.

Norrholm, S. D., and Ressler, K. J. 2009. "Genetics of Anxiety and Trauma-Related Disorders." *Neuroscience* 164(1): 272–287.

Norris, F., Foster, J., and Weisshaar, D. 2002. "The Epidemiology of Gender Differences in PTSD Across Developmental, Societal, and Research Contexts," in R. Kimerling, P. Ouimette, and J. Wolfe, eds., *Gender and PTSD*, 3–42. New York: Guilford.

Padgett, D., Gulcur, L., and Tsemberis, S. 2006. "Housing First Services for People Who Are Homeless with Co-Occurring Serious Mental Illness and Substance Abuse." *Research on Social Work Practice* 16(1): 74–78.

Palepu, A., Patterson, M., Moniruzzaman, K., Frankish, C., and Somers, J. 2013. "Housing First Improves Residential Stability in Homeless Adults with Concurrent Substance Dependence and Mental Disorders." *American Journal of Public Health* 103(2): E30–E36.

Parker, G. 2010. "Comoribidities in Bipolar Disorder: Models and Management." *Medical Journal of Australia* 193(4): S18–S20.

Patterson, M., Moniruzzaman, A., Palepu, A., Zabkiewicz, D., Frankish, C., Krausz, M., and Somers, J. 2013. "Housing First Improves Subjective Quality of Life Among Homeless Adults with Mental Illness: 12-Month Findings from a Randomized Controlled Trial in Vancouver, British Columbia." *Social Psychiatry and Psychiatric Epidemiology* 48(8): 1245–1259.

Pavokov, T., Lewis, D., and Lyons, J. 1989. "Psychiatric Diagnoses and Racial Bias: An Empirical Investigation." *Professional Psychology: Research and Practice* 20(6): 364–368.

Pedersen, D. 2002. "Political Violence, Ethnic Conflict, and Contemporary Wars: Broad Implications for Health and Social Well-Being." *Journal of Social Science and Medicine* 55(2): 175–190.

Perry, B., Neltner, M., and Allen, T. 2013. "A Paradox of Bias: Racial Differences in Forensic Psychiatric Diagnosis and Determinations of Criminal Responsibility." *Race and Social Problems* 5(4): 239–249.

Phelan, J. C., and Link, B. G. 2004. "Fear of People with Mental Illnesses: The Role of Personal and Impersonal Contact and Exposure to Threat or Harm." *Journal of Health and Social Behavior* 45(1): 68–80.

———. 2011. "The Stigma of Mental Illness and Psychiatric Disorders," in C. D. Bryant, ed., *The Routledge Handbook of Deviant Behavior*, 572–579. New York: Routledge.

Pickersgill, M. D. 2013. "Debating DSM-5: Diagnosis and the Sociology of Critique." *Journal of Medical Ethics*, 40: 521–525.

Pressman, J. D. 1997. "Psychiatry and Its Origins." *Bulletin of Historical Medicine* 71: 129–139.

Rayburn, N., Wenzel, S., Elliott, M., Hambarsoomian, K., Marshall, G., and Tucker, J. 2005. "Trauma, Depression, Coping, and Mental Health Service Seeking Among Impoverished Women." *Journal of Consulting and Clinical Psychology* 73(4): 667–677.

Read, J., Perry, B. D., Moskowitz, A., and Connolly, J. 2001. "The Contribution of Early Traumatic Events to Schizophrenia in Some Patients: A Traumagenic Neurodevelopmental Model." *Psychiatry* 64(4): 319–345.

Reilly, J., Ayis, S., Ferrier, I., Jones, S., and Thomas, S. 2000. "QTc-Interval Abnormalities and Psychotropic Drug Therapy in Psychiatric Patients." *Lancet* 355: 1048–1052.

Reynolds, G., and Kirk, S. 2010. "Metabolic Side Effects of Antipsychotic Drug Treatment—Pharmacological Mechanisms." *Pharmacology and Therapeutics* 125(1): 169–179.

Rhodes, A., Goering, P., To, T., and Williams, J. 2002. "Gender and Outpatient Mental Health Service Use." *Social Science and Medicine* 54: 1–10.

Rimke, H., and Brock, D. 2012. "The Culture of Therapy: Psychocentrism in Everyday Life," in M. Thomas, R. Raby, and D. Brock, eds., *Power and Everyday Practices*, 182–202. Toronto, ON: Nelson.

Robertson, M., and Winkleby, M. 1996. "Mental Health Problems of Homeless Women and Differences Across Subgroups." *American Review of Public Health* 17: 311–336.

Roe, C., McNamara, A., and Motheral, B. 2002. "Gender- and Age-Related Prescription Drug Use Patterns." *Annals of Pharmacotherapy* 36(1): 30–39.

Rogler, L. H 1997. "Making Sense of Historical Changes in the Diagnostic and Statistical Manual of Mental Disorders: Five Propositions." *Journal of Health and Social Behavior* 38(1): 9–20.

Rose, N. 1998. *Inventing Our Selves: Psychology, Power, and Personhood.* Cambridge: Cambridge University Press.

———. 2003. "Neurochemical Selves." *Society* 41(1): 46–59.

———. 2007. *The Politics of Life Itself: Biomedicine, Power, and Subjectivity in the Twenty-First Century*. Princeton: Princeton University Press.

Routh, D., and King, K. 1972. "Social Class Bias in Clinical Judgment." *Journal of Consulting and Clinical Psychology* 38(2): 202–207.

Rutter, M. 1987. "Psychosocial Resilience and Protective Mechanisms." *American Journal of Orthopsychiatry* 57: 316–331.

Rylko-Bauer, B., and Farmer, P. 2002. "Managed Care or Managed Inequality? A Call for Critiques of Market-Based Medicine." *Medical Anthropology Quarterly* 16: 476–502.

Sadow, D., and Ryder, M. 2008. "Reducing Stigmatizing Attitudes Held by Future Health Professionals: The Person Is the Message." *Psychological Services* 5(4): 362–372.

Scull, A. 2011. *Madness: A Very Short Introduction.* Oxford: Oxford University Press.

Seeman, M. 2012. "Antipsychotic-Induced Somnolence in Mothers with Schizophrenia." *Psychiatric Quarterly* 83: 83–89.

Sethi, K., Ed. 2004. *Drug-Induced Movement Disorders.* New York: Marcel Dekker.

Sexton, T. 2003, August 12. "Paxil Brings Suicidal Thoughts: Paxil May Have Undesirable Emotional Side Effects on Young People." *Psychology Today.* https://www.psychologytoday.com/articles/200908/paxil-brings-suicidal-thoughts (accessed September 13, 2015).

Simons, R., and Whitbeck, L. 1991. "Sexual Abuse as a Precursor to Prostitution and Victimization Among Adolescent and Adult Homeless Women." *Journal of Family Issues* 12(3): 361–379.

Singer, M. 2004. "The Social Origins and Expressions of Illness." *British Medical Bulletin* 69(1): 9–19.

Sismondo, S. 2007. "Ghost Management: How Much of the Medical Literature Is Shaped Behind the Scenes by the Pharmaceutical Industry?" *PLoS Medicine* 4(9).

Smith, K. 2015. "'Just Surviving': Domestic Work as a Form of Structural Violence in Sistren Theatre Collective's *Domestick.*" *Women's History Review* 24(3): 351–371.

Snow, D. A., and Anderson, L. 1993. *Down on Their Luck: A Study of Homeless Street People.* Berkeley: University of California Press.

Snow, N., and Austin, J. 2009. "Community Treatment Orders: The Ethical Balancing Act in Community Mental Health." *Journal of Psychiatric and Mental Health Nursing* 16: 177–186.

Snowden, L. 2003. "Bias in Mental Health Assessment and Intervention: Theory and Evidence." *American Journal of Public Health* 93(2): 239–243.

Sorenson, S., and Siegel, J. 1992. "Gender, Ethnicity, and Sexual Assault: Findings from a Los Angeles Study." *Journal of Social Issues* 48: 93–104.

Stein, J., Leslie, M., and Nyamathi, A. 2002. "Relative Contributions of Parent Substance Use and Childhood Maltreatment to Chronic Homelessness, Depression, and Substance Abuse Problems Among Homeless Women: Mediating Roles of Self-Esteem and Abuse in Adulthood." *Child Abuse and Neglect* 26(10): 1011–1027.

Stergiopoulos, V., Rouleau, K., and Yoder, S. 2007. "Shelter-Based Collaborative Mental Health Care for the Homeless." *Psychiatric Times* 24(8): 23–28.

Tam, T., Zlotnick, C., and Bradley, K. 2008. "The Link Between Homeless Women's Mental Health and Service System Use." *Psychiatric Services* 59(9): 1004–1010.

Tang, S. S. S., and Freyd, J. J. 2012. "Betrayal Trauma and Gender Differences in Posttraumatic Stress," *Psychological Trauma: Theory, Research, Practice, and Policy* 4(5): 469–478.

Tasca, C., Rapetti, M., Carta, M., and Fadda, B. 2012. "Women and Hysteria in the History of Mental Health." *Clinical Practice and Epidemiology in Mental Health* 8: 110–119.

Tedeschi, R., and Calhoun, L. 1995. *Trauma and Transformation: Growing in the Aftermath of Suffering*. Thousand Oaks, CA: Sage.

———. 1996. "The Posttraumatic Growth Inventory: Measuring the Positive Legacy of Trauma." *Journal of Traumatic Stress* 9(4): 455–471.

Tolin, D., and Foa, E. 2006. "Sex Differences in Trauma and Posttraumatic Stress Disorder: Quantitative Review of 25 Years of Research." *Psychological Bulletin* 132(6): 959–992.

Trollor, J., Chen, X., and Sachdev, P. 2009. "Neuroleptic Malignant Syndrome Associated with Atypical Antipsychotic Drugs." *CNS Drugs* 23(6): 477–492.

Tsai, J., Mares, A., and Rosenheck, R. 2010. "A Multisite Comparison of Supported Housing for Chronically Homeless Adults: Housing First Versus 'Residential Treatment First.'" *Psychiatric Services* 63(5): 427–434.

Tsemberis, S., Gulcar, L., and Nakae, M. 2004. "Housing First, Consumer Choice, and Harm Reduction for Homeless Individuals with a Dual Diagnosis." *American Journal of Public Health* 94(4): 651–656.

Tsuang, M. 2000. "Schizophrenia: Genes and Environment." *Biological Psychiatry* 47(3): 210–220.

Tyler, K., Melander, L., and Almazan, E. 2010. "Self Injurious Behavior Among Homeless Young Adults: A Social Stress Analysis." *Social Science and Medicine* 70(2): 269–276.

Ullman, S., Filipas, H., Townsend, S., and Starzynski, L. 2007. "Psychosocial Correlates of PTSD Symptom Severity in Sexual Assault Survivors." *Journal of Traumatic Stress* 20(5): 821–831.

Ungar, M. 2013. "Resilience, Trauma, Context, and Culture." *Trauma, Violence, and Abuse* 14(3): 255–266.

Walsh, B., Seidman, S., Sysko, R., and Gould, M. 2002. "Placebo Response in Studies of Major Depression: Variable, Substantial, and Growing." *JAMA* 287(14): 1840–1847.

Wang P., Lane M., Olfson M., Pincus, H., Wells, K., and Kessler, R. 2005. "Twelve-Month Use of Mental Health Services in the United States." *Archives of General Psychiatry* 62: 629–640.

Watanabe, J., Suzuki, Y., and Someya, T. 2013. "Lipid Effects of Psychiatric Medication." *Current Atherosclerosis Reports* 15(1): 292–298.

Wenzel, S., Koegel, P., and Gelberg, L. 2000. "Antecedents of Physical and Sexual Victimization Among Homeless Women: A Comparison to Homeless Men." *American Journal of Community Psychology* 28(3): 367–390.

Whitney, N., and Glazier, R. 2004. "Factors Affecting Medication Adherence Among the Homeless: A Qualitative Study of Patients' Perspectives." *University of Toronto Medical Journal* 82(1): 6–9.

Widiger, T. 1998. "Sex Biases in the Diagnoses of Personality Disorder." *Journal of Personality Disorders* 12: 95–118.

Wilson, P. T., and Spitzer, R. L. 1968. "Major Changes in Psychiatric Nomenclature: Reconciling Existing Psychiatric Medical Records with the New American Psychiatric Association *Diagnostic and Statistical Manual of Mental Disorders*." *Hospital and Community Psychiatry* 19(6): 169–174.

Wurtzel, E. 1994. *Prozac Nation: Young and Despressed in America*. New York: Penguin Books.

Yeater, E., Austin, J., Green, M., and Smith, J. 2010. "Coping Mediates the Relationship Between Posttraumatic Stress Disorder (PTSD) Symptoms and Alcohol Use in Homeless, Ethnically Diverse Women: A Preliminary Study." *Psychological Trauma: Theory, Research, Practice, and Policy* 2(4): 307–310.

Zizek, S. 2008. *Violence: Six Sideways Reflections*. New York: Picodor.

Index

About the Book

Despite widespread recognition that the majority of homeless women suffer from severe mental and emotional trauma, our healthcare system has essentially left them untreated—other than to mask their symptoms with psychiatric drugs. Why? And what can be done about it? Addressing this issue, Laura Huey and Rose Ricciardelli not only present an integrated analysis of the ways that the system is failing homeless women, but also propose a sensible alternative to the status quo.

Laura Huey is associate professor of sociology at the University of Western Ontario. She is author of *Negotiating Demands: The Politics of Skid Row Policing* and *Invisible Victims: Homelessness and the Growing Security Gap*. **Rose Ricciardelli** is associate professor of sociology at Memorial University of Newfoundland. She is author of *Surviving Incarceration Inside Canadian Prisons*.